8/17

THE INDIVIDUAL INCOME TAX
AND ECONOMIC GROWTH

THE INDIVIDUAL
INCOME TAX
AND ECONOMIC GROWTH

An International Comparison

France, Germany, Italy, Japan,

United Kingdom, United States

by Vito Tanzi

The Johns Hopkins Press
Baltimore

TO MADELEINE
TO MY PARENTS

PREFACE

Several years ago it was fashionable to ascribe the slower growth rates of the United States and the United Kingdom vis-à-vis European countries to their greater reliance on direct taxation. This assumption, however, was only examined in general terms—that is, limited to such general categories as direct versus indirect taxes. It seemed to me at the time that differences among specific parts of the tax systems might be as important in determining growth rates as differences in total tax structure, and I therefore decided to undertake a systematic comparison of the personal income tax systems of the six major industrial countries. This study, which required an enormous effort to obtain the necessary data, was presented as my doctoral dissertation to Harvard University in 1966. The data collected for the dissertation have formed the basis for this book.

It would be impossible to thank everyone who has assisted me with useful comments and suggestions or with collection of data. My greatest professional debt is to Otto Eckstein, who is also responsible for my interest in public finance. Special thanks also go to Richard A. Musgrave for his comments on the original work. I would like to acknowledge the help given me by the various embassies and by the Joint Library of the International Monetary Fund and the International Bank for Reconstruction and Development. Without the facilities of that library this study would not have been possible. I would also like to thank the members of the Joint Tax Program of the OAS-IDB with whom I was associated during part of the writing of this book, and Charles T. Stewart, Clay McCuistion, Noboru Tanabe, Ichizo Miyamoto, and Teruo Hirao.

This acknowledgment would constitute a great injustice if I did not mention my wife Madeleine. Words cannot express my gratitude to her. Besides typing the manuscript, she provided the essential moral support in an always patient and cheerful way.

Washington, D.C.   Vito Tanzi

CONTENTS

TABLES

LIST OF ILLUSTRATIONS

THE INDIVIDUAL INCOME TAX
AND ECONOMIC GROWTH

INTRODUCTION

TAX STRUCTURE AND ECONOMIC GROWTH

Many economic discussions in the last few years have placed considerable emphasis on economic growth. Growth has acquired a prominence and status comparable to that of more traditional economic objectives, such as price stability and full employment. This emphasis represents a departure from both neoclassical economics, with its insistence on general equilibrium and allocation of resources in a predominantly static setting, and Keynesian economics, with its insistence on the short run and full employment. We live now in a post-Keynesian world where the retort that "in the long run we are dead" no longer justifies a lack of concern for dynamic factors. Besides, it has become obvious that several short-run objectives, such as employment and balance of payments, are not independent of the long-run performance of the economy.

With the new emphasis, the tax systems of the industrial countries could not fail to attract considerable attention. This interest has been stimulated because these countries have experienced different rates of growth and have relied on fiscal systems which are structurally different. Economists have tried to link the so-called economic miracles of countries such as France, Italy, and, to a lesser extent, Germany to the fact that these countries rely, or have relied, heavily on indirect forms of taxation for their revenues. Similarly, it has been maintained that the slower rate of growth of the United States and the United Kingdom may have been the direct consequence of their excessive reliance on direct taxation.[1] In those discussions, little attempt was made at trying to define precisely what is meant by direct and indirect taxes. Such a distinction could be based on different criteria, and each of these

---

[1] It must be pointed out that since the tax cut of 1964 and the boom that followed, the tone of the pertinent writing has changed substantially. It is interesting to point out that the boom took place in the face of a basically unchanged structure of the tax system.

would give a specific classification which might, or might not, be consistent with that given by a different criterion.[2]

Some of these countries—particularly France and Italy—have had basically the same tax systems for several decades. Although their recent performance has been good, the same cannot be said for that of their past. In fact, the hypothesis has been put forward by some authors that the successful performance of the past decade has been primarily a consequence of a poor past performance.[3]

Another serious deficiency in these discussions has been the excessive emphasis on the *structures* of the tax systems as distinguished from the *level* of taxation. This attitude seems to be unjustified because, given the same tax structure (however this is defined), various *levels* of taxation will affect the countries differently.[4] However, a consideration of the level of taxation naturally implies that the *use* of the tax revenues should also be analyzed; but this produces a problem of enormous proportions.

The comparison of tax systems is not simple, and it is unlikely that broad classifications, such as those limited to direct versus indirect taxes, will provide sufficient information for reaching valid conclusions. It is likely, however, that differences within the system of direct taxation may be very important with respect to growth.[5] There may be specific characteristics of a direct tax of a country which may make it more of an obstacle to growth than a similar tax in another country. It is necessary, therefore, to disaggregate the tax systems and analyze the taxes one by one.

OBJECTIVE OF STUDY

The individual income tax was selected for detailed study because it is the most important of the direct taxes and because many tax experts think that it has been overemphasized in the English-speaking countries. I have decided to

---

[2]Ursula Hicks, "The Terminology of Tax Analysis," *Readings in the Economics of Taxation*, ed. Richard A. Musgrave and Carl S. Shoup (Homewood, Ill.: R. D. Irwin, Inc., 1959); Otto Eckstein, "Indirect Versus Direct Taxes: Implications for Stability Investment," *Excise Tax Compendium* (Washington, D. C.: G.P.O., 1964), Part I, p. 44.

[3]See, for example, Angus Maddison, *Economic Growth in the West* (New York: The Twentieth Century Fund, 1964), chap. ii; and John Knapp and Kenneth Lomax, "Britain's Growth Performance: The Enigma of the 1950's," *Lloyds Bank Review,* October 1964.

[4]In the recent analyses of the concept of "fiscal drag," the emphasis is on the *level* of taxation rather than on the structure. If fiscal factors played a leading role in the post-1963 boom, it was the income effect of the tax cut, rather than the change in the structure, that was most important.

[5]See Fritz Neumark, comment on paper by Otto Eckstein (assisted by Vito Tanzi), "Comparison of European and United States Tax Structures and Growth Implications," N.B.E.R. and The Brookings Institution *The Role of Direct and Indirect Taxes in the Federal Revenue System* (Princeton: Princeton University Press, 1964), p. 287.

compare and analyze this tax for the most important industrial countries of the noncommunist world—France, Germany, Italy, Japan, the United Kingdom, and the United States.

It would be ideal if one could ask a simple question (such as, which country had a personal income tax that was most harmful to the growth of the economy?) and make a frontal attack in trying to answer it. But this is not realistic, and I have concentrated on a few basic issues and dealt with them individually.

First is the issue of sacrifice or burden connected with individual income taxation. It has been argued that the individual income taxes of the United States and the United Kingdom have imposed very heavy burdens on their taxpayers with resultant adverse effects on individual incentive. The basis for this contention has been the comparison of the ratios of the individual income taxes to the national incomes of the countries. This question of tax burdens or sacrifices will be analyzed in detail by using different concepts of burden and by analyzing the relationship between the income subjected to taxation and the national income.

Second, the relationship between the individual income tax and the propensity of the household sector to save, is examined. I have concentrated on the aspects of the individual income taxes (such as, de facto progressivity and taxation of high income groups, different treatment of various kinds of incomes, and specific legal provisions for encouraging saving) which are assumed to influence personal saving.

Third, I examine the relationship of the individual income taxes of these countries to their economic growth.

Each of these questions is interesting in itself; however, it is jointly that they explain the influence of the individual income tax on the performance of the economy. If a given country had a "burden" which, regardless of the concept used, was heavier than that of the other countries; if this country placed an especially heavy tax on higher income groups and the incomes from business and investment as compared with those from wages and salaries; if it did nothing to prevent the revenues from the individual income tax from growing faster than the national income; then, one would be justified in concluding that, relative to the other countries, the individual income tax of this country was a negative influence on economic growth.

A few words about the limitations of this study are in order. It was impossible to analyze the entire tax systems of the six countries, and I have therefore considered the individual income taxes by themselves, apart from the context of the tax systems as a whole. Secondly, because of difficulties in obtaining data, I could not integrate as much as I would have liked the nominal with the structural characteristics of the different income tax systems. Finally, owing to the separate consideration of the income taxes, the discussion of equity issues was necessarily limited.

IMPORTANCE OF THE INDIVIDUAL INCOME TAXES

The scope and importance of the individual income tax differ from country to country. Since this tax will be considered in isolation, it seems wise to start with a general sketch of the countries' tax systems and a clear idea of the relative importance of the individual income tax.[6]

France depends on indirect taxation for between 70 and 75 per cent of her revenues. Until a couple of years ago, the system was becoming even more dependent on indirect taxes, but recently this trend seems to have been reversed. The individual income tax has accounted for only about 13 per cent of the total tax revenue compared with the 35 per cent obtained from the value added taxes.[7]

The role of the individual income tax is much more significant in Germany. It has accounted for about 35 per cent of the total national tax revenues in the last few years. This share has been increasing from 27.5 per cent in 1956. Germany also has a very productive general sales tax, the turnover tax, which has been accounting for about 25 per cent of the total revenues of the national government. Apart from these two taxes, the most important levies are: the corporation tax, which normally amounts to about 10 per cent of the total revenues; the tobacco tax, which, though still very important, has been losing ground; and the mineral oil tax, which has been increasing in importance over the years. These last two taxes have normally been as productive as the corporation tax.[8]

The revenue system of Italy, like that of France, is greatly dependent on indirect forms of taxation. Over 75 per cent of all tax revenues are obtained in this manner. The *Ricchezza Mobile* is the most important among the direct taxes; it accounts for 14 to 16 per cent of the total tax revenue of the central government of Italy. The *Ricchezza Mobile* cannot be considered strictly an *individual* income tax since the most important of the schedules, B, concerns

---

[6]For a concise description of the individual income taxes, see Chapter II. For a brief description of the systems of the four European countries, see Vito Tanzi, "Notes on European Tax Systems," appendix to Otto Eckstein, "Comparison of European and United States Tax Structures and Growth Implications," *op. cit.,* pp. 251-85. For Japan, see Taizo Hayashi, *Guide to Japanese Taxes, 1965* (Tokyo: Zaikei Shoho Sha, 1965). For more authoritative studies, the volumes of the Harvard Law School World Tax Series should be consulted.

[7]For detail, see Institut National de la Statistique et des Etudes Economiques, *Tableaux de l'Economie Française, 1966* (Paris: 1966), p. 295.

[8]For detail, see Germany, Deutsche Bundesbank, *Monthly Report.* At the time of writing this study, Germany was considering changing the turnover tax into a value-added tax.

the income of enterprises regardless of their juridical form. Another tax on individual income is the *Imposta Complementare sul Reddito Complessivo,* a tax on global income. The importance of this tax is really minor, accounting for only 2 to 3 per cent of the total tax revenues.

The most important of Italy's indirect taxes is the *Imposta Generale sulla Entrata* (I.G.E.) which is a turnover tax of a cascade type. This is really the cornerstone of the tax system of Italy, accounting for as much as the direct taxes combined (around 21 per cent of the total). Of the remaining indirect taxes, two are of major importance, rivaling in magnitude the *Ricchezza Mobile.* These two taxes are the mineral oils tax (which yields about 14 per cent of the total) and the tobacco tax (which accounted for 14.6 per cent in 1954-55 and 8.8 per cent in 1965).[9]

In Japan, the individual income tax has accounted for between 20 and 35 per cent of the total national taxes. Since 1950 its relative importance has been declining, while that of the corporate income tax has been increasing. These two taxes combined amounted to over half of the total revenue (57.5 per cent in 1964). The liquor tax was also of particular importance, providing 17.1 per cent of the total in 1955 and 11.3 per cent in 1964. While the gasoline tax has been increasing in importance (yielding 2.7 per cent in 1955 and 7.5 per cent in 1964), the sugar tax has been decreasing from 5.1 per cent in 1955 to .8 per cent in 1964.[10] The exceptional rate of growth of the Japanese economy has induced the government to adopt a "tax-cut policy" in order to limit the natural growth in revenues.

The tax system of the United Kingdom is heavily dependent on income taxes which account for more than half of all the tax receipts of the central government (50.3 per cent in 1963). The total individual income tax in 1963 (£2,507 million) was 37.3 per cent of all the tax revenues (£6,727 million). The remaining 13 per cent came from taxes on the income of corporations and from profits taxes. The most important of the other taxes are those on tobacco (13.2 per cent of the total), on hydrocarbon oils (8.5 per cent), and on beer (3.8 per cent). The United Kingdom also has a general sales tax which is collected at the wholesale level. The revenue from this tax was 8.4 per cent of the total in 1963.[11]

Table I-1 shows the importance of the individual income tax in the gross national products and in the total tax revenues of each country. It is clearly predominant in the United States, where it accounts for over 50 per cent of

---

[9]For detail, see Ministero delle Finanze, *L'Attività Tributaria nel 1965* (Rome: Istituto Poligrafico dello Stato, 1966), p. 21.

[10]See Japan, Ministry of Finance, Tax Bureau, *An Outline of Japanese Taxes, 1964* (Tokyo: 1965), p. 14.

[11]See Great Britain, Central Statistical Office, *National Income and Expenditure, 1964* (London: H.M.S.O., 1965).

TABLE I-1. SHARE OF THE INDIVIDUAL INCOME TAX
IN THE GNP AND IN THE TAX REVENUES OF THE
CENTRAL GOVERNMENTS OF SIX COUNTRIES, 1963

Country	% of tax revenues	% of GNP
France	12.5	2.72
Germany	35.0	7.55
Italy	16.2	3.34
United Kingdom	37.3	8.86
Japan	25.0	3.01
United States	55.1	8.13

Sources: For the United States: U.S., Council of Economic Advisers, *Economic Report of the President* (Washington, D.C.: G.P.O., 1966). For the other countries: O.E.C.D., *National Accounts Statistics, 1954-1964* (Paris: O.E.C.D., March 1966); and the national sources cited above.

the revenues of the federal government, and in the United Kingdom and Germany, where it accounts for about one-third of total revenues. In Japan, it amounts to about 25 per cent, while in Italy and France it is much lower.

The inclusion of the local governments would have the effect of lowering the percentage for the United States and bringing it much closer to that for Germany and the United Kingdom. On the other hand, if employees' contributions to social security had been considered as individual income taxes and included in the calculations of Table I-1, the figures for Italy and France would have been much higher.

With regard to the percentage of the individual income taxes in the gross national product of the six countries, the countries are grouped around two means: the first, comprised of Germany, the United Kingdom, and the United States, has a mean percentage of around 8 per cent; France, Italy, and Japan have a mean percentage of around 3 per cent. A major objective of this study will be to explain the reasons for these differences.

II

LEGAL STRUCTURE OF THE PERSONAL INCOME TAXES IN FIVE INDUSTRIAL COUNTRIES

This chapter provides a brief discussion of the personal income tax legislation of the five foreign countries under consideration. It is presented as a short informal background introduction and can be bypassed by anyone not interested in the legal aspects. More definitive statements can be found in the volumes put out by the Program in International Taxation sponsored by the Harvard Law School. The U.S. system is discussed in great detail in a recently published book by Richard Goode.[1]

FRANCE

General Background

The personal income tax was introduced in France in 1917, but its importance in the French fiscal system has been rather limited. Until the fiscal reform of December 28, 1959, there were two distinct taxes on income. The first was a proportional tax (*la taxe proportionnelle*) on each of the income categories with some exceptions, while the second was a progressive tax (*surtaxe progressive*) on the global income. Article 1 of the law of December 28, 1959 eliminated these two taxes and replaced them with a single, progressive tax on total personal incomes (*impôt sur le revenu des personnes physiques*). Temporarily, however, for reason of revenue needs, a proportional tax (*taxe complémentaire*) was imposed to be repealed in 1965.

Taxable Income

Taxable income is the combined income of the head of the household, his wife, and dependent children, and is reported according to categories which reflect the origin of that income. The total income is combined and the tax is levied on it, but some discrimination still remains in the treatment of each particular category. The income categories are the following:

[1] Richard Goode, *The Individual Income Tax* (Washington, D. C.: The Brookings Institution, 1964).

7

1. Income from land and buildings (*revenus fonciers*). This includes the net income from buildings. In the case of owner-occupied houses, a rent is imputed to them but many deductions are allowed. These include all expenses for repairs as well as 30 per cent of gross income (20 per cent for rural property) for depreciation.

2. Industrial and trading profits (*bénéfices industriels et commerciaux*). These incomes may be taxed according to the actual reported income (*bénéfice réel*) or, with some limitations, according to the "normal" (*forfait*) assessed profits of the enterprise.

3. Remuneration of managing partners.

4. Agricultural profits (*bénéfices de l'exploitation agricole*). These, too, are normally assessed by the administration (*régime du forfait*). The assessment is obtained by multiplying the estimated peracre income, as published yearly by the authority, by the area under cultivation. Thus the income reported is the assessed rather than the actual one. If there is cause, however, either the taxpayer or the administration may opt for the *régime de bénéfice réel.*

5. Wages, salaries, and life pensions (*traitements, salaires, pensions et rentes viagères*). The taxable income is obtained by deducting the following from gross income: family allowances; earnings retained by the employers for purposes of pensions; payments for social security; 10 per cent of the income for occupational expenses. Twenty per cent of the income thus obtained is also deducted. These deductions apply exclusively to wages and salaries, and thus special treatment is provided for such incomes.

6. Nontrading profits (*bénéfices non commerciaux*). This category includes, among others, the incomes from professional activities.

7. Investment income *(revenus des capitaux mobiliers)*. These are incomes from dividends, stocks, bonds, deposits, etc. Since the reform of 1959, the law has established a withholding tax at the source fixed at: 12 per cent for the interests from negotiable obligations emitted in France;[2] 24 per cent for dividends and other *revenus mobiliers.* The tax which is thus paid can be imputed in the general tax payment of the taxpayer.

The French tax legislation assumes that the global income reported by a family cannot be less than that expected by the standard of living of that family. Whenever the income is less, the tax authority replaces the declared income with an imputed income, but this occurs only when the imputed income exceeds F15,000.

Deductions and Exemptions

Apart from those mentioned above, French law allows the following deductions: some business losses can be carried forward; interest paid

---

[2]For bonds issued after January 1, 1965 the rate has been reduced to 10 per cent.

(subject to several restrictions); some pensions; the *taxe complémentaire;* social security contributions; payments for unemployment insurance; some payments for premiums on life insurance; contributions (up to .5 per cent of taxable income) to charities, educational and scientific organizations, etc.; and the share of income saved and invested in construction.

Exempted from the tax are incomes from interest on government and other public securities and incomes of taxpayers who benefit mainly from wages, salaries, life annuities, pensions, and similar incomes and whose total income does not exceed the minimum, interprofessional guaranteed income.

Treatment of Families

For purposes of taxation, the total income of the family is divided into parts according to the following plan.

single	1 part
married with no children	2 parts
divorced (or single) with one dependent	2 parts
married or widow with one dependent	2.5 parts
single or divorced with two dependent children	2.5 parts
married or widow with two children	3 parts

For each additional child, a half part is granted. The family income is split among the parts, and each part is taxed separately on its share of the total income. Because of this, the progressivity of the income tax is substantially reduced with the increase in the size of the family.

Capital Gains

France does not have any capital gains tax. However, in the case of the sale of land and buildings within five years after the date of acquisition, any gains are taxed at a minimum rate of 15 per cent. The taxpayer may claim exemption if he is able to prove that there was no intent to speculate. Of course, people who engage regularly in real estate are taxed with the regular income tax rates. No tax is paid if the property is held for more than five years within certain limitations.[3]

[3]International Bureau of Fiscal Documentation, *European Taxation,* September 1965, p. 234.

Rates

The rates at which each part of the global taxable income of 1965 was taxed are shown below.

Income Brackets in Francs	Rate in Per Cent
0 - 2,400	5
2,401 - 4,500	15
4,501 - 7,600	20
7,601 - 11,250	25
11,251 - 18,000	35
18,001 - 36,000	45
36,001 - 72,000	55
above 72,001	65

Once the tax is calculated with these rates, it is reduced by 5 per cent of the wages and salaries included in the computation of taxable income if the latter have been subjected to the *versement forfaitaire.* The tax is not collected whenever it does not exceed F80 per part. When it is between F80 and F240 the tax liability is reduced by half the difference between F240 times the number of parts and the tax which has been calculated. The tax due is increased by 5 per cent whenever the taxable income exceeds F45,000 regardless of the number of parts.

Method of Payment

Only incomes paid to people who do not reside in France and the incomes from investments of funds are withheld at the source. All the other taxpayers complete a form with the relevant information on their income and mail it to the tax authorities who compute the tax and inform the taxpayers how much they owe. The form must be filed by March 1 of the year following that in which the income has been received. The payments follow much later.

Complementary Tax

This tax which was imposed for temporary budgetary needs is not a progressive tax and is much less comprehensive than the *Impôt sur les revenus des personnes physiques;* it does not apply to wages and salaries, pensions and annuities, investment income, and in certain cases income from independent professions. Only incomes in excess of either F4,400 (nontrading profits) or F3,000 (incomes from land, industrial, and trading profits and some others) are taxed. The complementary tax is deductible from the progressive income tax. The rate of this tax was 6 per cent in 1965.

GERMANY

General Background

The German personal income tax is not, strictly speaking, a federal tax but a tax which is apportioned between the Länder and the federal government according to shares which have averaged around 65 per cent for the former and 35 per cent for the latter. The shares are established by law for each fiscal year.[4]

The German income tax in its present form is a direct descendant of the Prussian income tax of June 19, 1906, which was progressive but with very low rates.[5] Those rates, however, were substantially increased between the two wars. In 1925 the tax became federal with a maximum rate of 39 per cent reached at an income of DM80,000. By 1934 it had reached 50 per cent for single taxpayers.[6]

Legally there are four income taxes in Germany today: the adjudicated income tax (*Einkommensteuer*), the wage and salary tax (*Lohnsteuer*), the tax on the return of financial capital (*Kapitalertragsteuer*), and the corporation tax (*Koeperschaftssteuer*). Of course, of these, only the first three are taxes on personal income.

Taxable Income

The law declares the following taxable: incomes from agriculture and forestry, industrial and commercial profits, incomes from liberal professions, incomes from wages and salaries, incomes from capital, rents, and others specified in the law.

General Exemptions and Deductions

Several receipts are exempted from the tax. The most important among them are: receipts from insurance for sickness and invalidism, unemployment compensation, capital indemnity for old-age insurance, old-age insurance receipts up to DM600, many other receipts from pensions, and interest received on public (federal and Länder) securities.

Deductions may be made (up to DM1,100 for the taxpayer and his spouse and DM500 for each dependent child) for interest payments, obligatory contributions for insurance against sickness and accidents connected with employment, and some life and real property insurance. The other main deductions are: contributions paid to saving institutions for construction; the

[4] These shares were: 38 per cent for 1953-54 and 1954-55, 33 1/3 per cent for 1955-56 to 1957-58; 35 per cent for 1958-59 on.

[5] Frederick G. Reuss, *Fiscal Policy for Growth without Inflation* (Baltimore: The Johns Hopkins Press, 1963), p. 82.

[6] *Ibid.*, p. 83.

church tax; the net wealth tax; the land tax and part of the equalization of burden tax; contributions paid in connection with the law on family allowances; contributions to charities and religious, educational, and scientific activities (up to 5 per cent of total income); and others (union dues, costs of tools, depreciation of houses, and automobile expenses of commuting to work).

Personal Deductions

The taxpayer may deduct DM1,680 for himself, DM1,680 for his spouse, DM1,200 for the first dependent child, DM1,680 for the second dependent child and DM1,800 for the third and each subsequent child.

For married taxpayers, splitting of income similar to that practiced in the United States is allowed. The system of joint returns without the possibility of splitting was in existence until June 1958 when it was found to be unconstitutional by the Supreme Constitutional Court.

There are additional deductions for special circumstances as follows: DM840 for unmarried people over fifty years of age, DM1,200 for single people with one dependent child, DM600 for all taxpayers over seventy, and DM1,200 for married couples when both are over seventy.

Rates

The rates of the income tax which were in effect from 1956 to 1964 were as follows: for the part of *taxable* income which did not exceed DM8,009 (DM16,016 for married couples), the rate was proportional and equal to 20 per cent; for the part of income between DM8,009 and DM110,039, the rate was progressive and varied from 20 to 60 per cent.

For the part of income which exceeded DM110,039 (or DM220,079 for married couples) the rate became proportional and was equal to 53 per cent. Within the range for which the tax was progressive, the progressivity was of a continuous kind. In other words, the tax did not jump from one bracket to the next; it increased smoothly. This is claimed to be an important advantage since it is not assumed to have the disincentive effect attributed to the staggered system prevalent in the United States and in the United Kingdom.

Starting with January 1, 1965, the rates have been changed slightly for reasons of basic economic policy. In fact, in 1958, 48 per cent of the income earners in Germany were exempted from the income tax; by 1963, the percentage had decreased to 25 per cent.

Capital Gains

Generally, capital gains, if held for a given period, are not taxed. However, what are mistakingly called "speculative transactions" are included in the taxable income of an individual. These are sales of real property or personal property (securities) held for less than a minimum period which is two years for the former and six months for the latter. Capital losses may be offset only against capital gains and may not be carried forward to future years or back to past years.

Method of Payment

Normally the taxpayer is required to make provisional payments, based on the amount of the tax paid the preceding year, on the 10th of March, June, September, and December. At the end of the fiscal year, the taxpayer is either reimbursed or he must pay the difference between the amount he has already paid and what he owes on the basis of the year's income.

In three cases, however, the tax is withheld at the source: (a) tax on wages and salaries (*Lohnsteuer*); (b) tax on revenues from financial investments (*Kapitalertragsteuer*), which is withheld at the rate of 25 per cent and which can be credited against the income tax; and (c) tax on incomes of managers of enterprises (*Aufsichtsratsteuer*).

Normally taxpayers whose income is obtained from wages and salaries are not required to submit any annual declaration.

ITALY

General Background

Of the countries considered in this study, Italy is probably the one which relies least on the taxation of personal income. The revenues from this tax *base* are quite small in spite of the fact that the Italian constitution states explicitly in article 53 that "everybody is required to contribute to the public expenditures in accordance with his contributing capacity. The tax system must follow criteria of progressivity."

Whether the Italian tax system is, in fact, progressive nobody really knows since there is no empirical study of this problem. In view of the very limited role of taxes on personal income, one can only guess that the system is not progressive.[7] If any effective progression does exist, it is to be found in the qualitative discrimination of incomes which treats incomes from work more favorably than income from capital (see below).

Formally, personal income is taxed first according to the schedule in which it falls (determined by the origin—i.e., from work, buildings, land, capital, etc.—of the income); then the income from all sources is combined and taxed as a whole.

[7]This is not to say that the impact of public finance (rather than the tax system) is not progressive, but this is a different issue. Anyway the constitution speaks of "tax system," not "public finance."

Schedular Taxes on Income

The "objective" or "real" taxes and the incomes to which they apply can be classified in two groups. The following taxes are in the first group:[8] tax on income from landowning (*imposta fondiaria or imposta sui terreni*), tax on income from buildings (*imposta sui fabbricati*), and tax on agricultural income (*imposta sul reddito agrario*).

The first two are taxes on income from real property, while the third is a tax on movable wealth and, therefore, strictly speaking belongs to the much more important group of the *Ricchezza Mobile*. The importance of these taxes is really minimal; the income imputed to them is normally much less than the actual income because the assessment (Catasto) of value is outdated.[9]

To the second group belongs the tax on income from movable wealth (*imposta sui redditi di ricchezza mobile*). This tax is made up of four very important taxes which reflect the schedules of movable income and are denoted by the letters A, B, C_1, and C_2.

Schedule A includes the tax on income from pure (movable) capital, which is income that requires no participation on the part of the income receiver and which is a fixed, rather than variable, entity. Therefore, schedule A includes incomes from bonds, bank deposits, saving accounts, and interest derived from loans and from certain insurance contracts. Income from government securities is tax exempt. Of the tax on the incomes in this schedule, only that on bonds is not greatly evaded since it is withheld at the source.

Before 1962, corporate securities were also supposed to be taxed with this schedule. However, it was almost impossible to ascertain the bearer so that these incomes were almost completely unreported. Since 1962, a withholding tax of 15 per cent has been applied.

Schedule B includes income from mixed capital and work (mainly enterprise income). This is income which cannot be included either in A (pure capital) or in C (labor income). This schedule includes income from executive work or, in general, work of an entrepreneurial nature. It also includes the income of the larger, nonincorporated businesses as well as that of incorporated businesses. In view of the inclusion of corporate profits, most of the revenues from the tax on these incomes cannot be considered to come from "personal" incomes.

[8]Charles K. Cobb, Jr. and Francesco Forte, *Taxation in Italy* (Cambridge, Mass.: Harvard Law School, 1964), pp. 15ff.

[9]See Francesco Forte, "Italy," N.B.E.R. and The Brookings Institution, *Foreign Tax Policies and Economic Growth* (Washington, D. C.: N.B.E.R. and The Brookings Institution, 1966).

Schedule C refers to income from work and is subdivided into two components C_1 and C_2. C_1 includes income from independent work, liberal professions, artisan activities, and similar activities; it also includes income from small enterprises. C_2 includes income from wages and salaries.

With the passing of time, although these taxes have remained "real" or "objective" in the sense that the economic situation of the taxpayer is not taken into consideration, they have lost their character of strict proportionality. Apart from schedule A, the reform of 1965 has rendered them decisively progressive at least on paper.

Progressive Tax on Global Income (Imposta Complementare Progressiva sul Reddito Globale). The individual's combined income from all taxable sources forms the basis on which this tax is applied. Contrary to the schedular taxes, this is a *personal* tax in so far as it takes into consideration the status of an individual. It is progressive with marginal rates reaching, since 1962,[10] 65 per cent on an income exceeding 500 million lire. The progression is continuous like the German one.

The minimum gross income subjected to the tax was raised in 1964 from 720,000 lire to 960,000 lire per year. That is, gross incomes which are smaller than the minimum taxable income of 960,000 lire are not taxed. Whenever the income exceeds 960,000 lire, after subtracting other taxes such as *Ricchezza Mobile, imposta di famiglia,* and other deductions such as insurance premiums, the following deductions may be made: 240,000 lire for the taxpayer himself; 50,000 for his wife and each subsequent dependent; 190,000 lire whenever both husband and wife receive incomes subjected to category C_2 (compensation for baby-sitting and similar expenses); and 20 per cent (not exceeding 360,000 lire) from incomes subjected to the schedular tax C_2 (incomes from dependent work).

Capital Gains

Except for gains of professional speculators, which are taxed according to schedule B of the *Ricchezza Mobile* and are included in the complementary income tax, capital gains in Italy are not taxed.

JAPAN

General Background

The introduction of the personal income tax in Japan dates as far back as 1887 when a global income tax was introduced with progressive rates ranging from 1 per cent to 3 per cent, and with a basic exemption granted to individuals. As one would expect, the role of this tax at that time was rather

[10]Law of April 4, 1962, No. 209.

limited (1.5 per cent of total tax revenues in 1888 compared to 53.8 per cent from the land tax). With the passing of time, its role has increased considerably. Its share of total tax revenues increased to 7.9 per cent in 1908, 20 per cent in 1921, 28.4 per cent in 1941, and 43.8 per cent in 1949.

In 1940 there was a basic reform of the income tax with the introduction of a corporation income tax, personal income tax schedules with different tax rates, and a 6 per cent withholding tax for employment income. This made 1,300,000 wage earners subject to the withholding. In 1947 the schedular system was replaced by a system of taxation of aggregate income.

Taxable Income

Individual taxable income is computed on a calendar year basis and is classified in ten categories (interest income, dividend income, employment income, etc.), but it is only the aggregate that is subjected to the tax. However, some forms of income (retirement and timber income and, in specified situations, interest and dividend income) are taxed separately.

Deductions and Exemptions

The taxpayer is entitled to a *basic* exemption of 120,000 yen and an additional 110,000 yen for his *spouse* when the spouse's income does not exceed 50,000 yen. The exemptions for dependents (other than the spouse) with not more than 50,000 yen of income each are as follows:

1. If an exemption has been provided for the spouse, it is 50,000 yen if the age of the dependent exceeds thirteen years, and 40,000 yen if it does not.

2. If no exemption is granted to the spouse, the exemption is 70,000 yen if there is only one dependent. Otherwise it is 70,000 yen for the first dependent over thirteen years of age; 50,000 yen for each other above thirteen years of age; 40,000 yen for each one younger than thirteen.

The main deductions allowed are: losses, due to acts of God, over 10 per cent of the total income; medical and dental expenses of over 5 per cent (up to 150,000 yen) of income; payments for social security contributions; premiums paid for life insurance (up to 35,000 yen) and for fire insurance.

Capital Gains

Capital gains are not taxed unless they arise in connection with professional speculations.

Rates

The net income, after exemptions and deductions, is taxed at rates of 8 to 75 per cent.

Method of Payment

In specified situations, Japanese income tax laws allow averaging for fluctuating incomes. Taxes on incomes from wages, salaries, interest, dividends, and other incomes specified by the law are withheld at the source. All other incomes are taxed by means of a self-assessment system.

UNITED KINGDOM

General Background

Income as the basis of taxation was introduced in Britain in 1799 when additional funds were needed in the war against France. In 1802, this tax was withdrawn for a few months but was reintroduced in 1803 at which time the income tax was enacted. In 1909 a forerunner of the present surtax (then called "supertax") was introduced with application limited to incomes above £5,000 and with a low rate (less than 3 per cent). The method of Pay-As-You-Earn (P.A.Y.E.) was introduced in 1943. In 1952 there was the last consolidation of the law concerning the taxation of income—the Income Tax Act. Since that time there have been many minor changes but no major ones.

Taxable Income

British tax legislation does not provide a definition of income but rather provides a classification of incomes, profits, or gains which must be subjected to the tax. The origin of this classification is found in the Income Tax Act of 1803. The classification, however, does not exhaust the possible sources of income since there is a catch-all category (paragraph VI of schedule D) which includes all the incomes not elsewhere classified. Up to 1964 taxable income also included the imputed rent of owner-occupied residences.

The incomes of individuals are classified according to schedules, depending on their economic origin. However, all schedules are taxed at the same rate so that, in spite of its appearance, the British income tax system is not schedular, like the Italian, but is rather similar to that of the United States or Germany. However, as it will be seen, some differentiation among kinds of incomes is accorded by specific reliefs for "earned" incomes.

The scope of the tax is very broad, applying to practically all incomes with the exception of some interest incomes. The year of assessment begins on the 6th of April.

The schedules are the following:

Schedule A. This schedule which used to include the incomes from the ownership of land, buildings, and "other hereditaments" and the imputed rent from owner-occupied property was suppressed by the Finance Act of 1963 and its income was transferred to schedule D.

Schedule B. It is unimportant and concerns income from the "occupation" of woodlands which are not exploited for commercial reasons.

Schedule C. This schedule pertains to interest on certain government securities (British and Commonwealth). The tax is withheld at the source whenever the interest payment exceeds £5.

Schedule D. Industrial, commercial, and agricultural profits, professional income, most interest payments, some occasional profits, gains from short-term speculations and rents are included in this schedule.

Schedule E. From the point of view of the revenue of income tax, this is the most important schedule, including incomes from offices, employment, or pensions. Practically all incomes received in connection with employment are taxable. Family allowances are similarly taxed and so are pensions in general. In this respect the British income tax differs from that of the continental countries. However, pensions for invalids, sickness pay, unemployment compensation, and some others are not taxed.

General Deductions

The following items fall in the category of general deductions:

1. Of professional expenses, only those which are "wholly, exclusively and necessarily" incurred by the employee in carrying out his functions are allowed to be deducted. This is a very restrictive requirement which was slightly relaxed by the Finance Act of 1958 which permitted the deduction of dues to professional organizations and subscription fees to professional journals.

2. Contributions to social security are deductible except for the part which goes to unemployment, sickness, and maternity premiums. Furthermore, two-fifths of the life insurance premiums (subject to limitations) and contributions by employees to a superannuation fund approved by the Inland Revenue are allowed a deduction.

3. Payments in kind are always taxable if given to people whose salary exceeds £2,000. They are not taxable in other cases.

4. Severance pay (indemnity for suspension of work) was not taxable until 1960 but it led to some abuses. Therefore, since 1960 it has been taxable for the excess over £5,000.

5. Charities are deductible if the taxpayer signs a deed obliging himself to make annual payments to recognized institutions for a period of over six years (pursuant to the Charities Act of 1960, more than 10,000 charities are registered).

Personal Deductions

Earned Income Relief. Earned income, which is accorded a special deduction, includes income from work as well as mixed income. Therefore, it is by no means limited to workers but includes wages, salaries, pensions, bonuses, directors' fees, business profits, benefits in kind, and income from patent rights. In this respect, it differs from the deductions permitted to income from wages and salaries by the French law. Nonearned incomes are specifically dividends, interests, rents, and profits for silent partners.

The earned income relief permits a certain proportion of the income—after all permissible expenses have been subtracted—to be deducted in order to get the assessable income. This relief for 1964-65 was equal to two-ninths of incomes up to £4,005 and one-ninth of incomes between £4,005 and £9,945. Thus, the limit is £1,550 while until 1957 it was £450. For married couples the deduction applies to the combined income and may not exceed £1,550.

Personal Relief. The allowance for single taxpayers is £200; for married taxpayers, it is £320. Whenever part of the family income is earned by the wife, two-sevenths of her income (up to £200) may be deducted.

Old Age Relief. Single taxpayers aged sixty-five or over, and married ones where either has reached this age, are not taxed if the income is £360 for the first and £575 for the latter. Further reductions are allowed for income above this level but below certain limits (two-ninths for incomes up to £200).

Small Income Relief. For incomes of any kind less than £450, two-ninths of the income can be deducted. For incomes between £450 and £680, the relief (since 1963-64) is half the excess over £450.

Child Relief. Whenever the child earns less than £115, relief is accorded as follows: £115 if the child is less than eleven years old; £140 if he is between eleven and sixteen; and £165 if he is over sixteen and a full-time student.

Other Reliefs. Additional allowances are granted for the following: housekeeper relief (£75), widows and other special cases (£40), and dependent relative relief (£75 per dependent).

Rate

The first £100 after all deductions are taxed at 20 per cent and the next £200 at 30 per cent. The taxable income above £300 is taxed at a standard rate, which was 38.75 per cent from 1959 until April 1965 and 41.25 per cent after that. The standard rate was 42.5 per cent for the period 1955-56 to 1958-59 and 45 per cent between 1953-54 and 1955-56.

Surtax. To assure progressivity of the income tax not only at low levels of income but also at high levels, the British system imposes a surtax on top of the standard rate. It was introduced in the Finance Act of 1907 and apart from changes in the rates it has not changed much since then.

The surtax makes the taxation of personal income in the United Kingdom the heaviest of any large country. Two reforms in the last few years have tried to mitigate its harshness. The first of these reforms was introduced by the Finance Act of 1957 which extended to the surtax many of the deductions which were allowed to the income tax. Some of these were the single allowance, the married allowance, child relief, housekeeping, and some others.

The second reform, that of 1961, was much more significant. The "earned income relief," which, as seen above, may total £1,550 was now allowed to the surtax in the same conditions as to the income tax. In addition, an "earnings allowance" was also allowed. This is equal to the excess of the earned income as reduced by the earned income relief over £2,000 subject to a maximum allowance of £2,000.

The advantages of these two reforms have accrued to "earned" incomes (i.e., incomes from work and mixed). They have not benefited incomes from investments (dividends, interest, rents, etc.) which represent a very large proportion of the incomes of people with high global incomes (about one half of incomes above £10,000 and two-thirds of incomes beyond £20,000). Because of these reforms, the surtax which applies to investment incomes above £2,000 does not become payable on earned income until it reaches about £5,000, the precise figure depending upon the personal allowances. The effect of the 1961 reform is seen clearly in the composition of total income subjected to the surtax for the years 1960-61 and 1961-62. In the first of these two fiscal years, earned income was 67 per cent higher than investment income (£1,265 compared to £760). In the second year, it was lower (£770 compared to £775).

The marginal rates for the surtax range from 10 per cent on the first £500 to 50 per cent on incomes above £13,000.

Capital Gains

Up to the enactment of the Finance Act of 1962, capital gains were generally not taxed unless they could be proved to be business incomes. The Finance Act of 1962 introduced a short-term capital gains tax, according to which assets acquired after April 10, 1962 would be subjected to the income, surtax, and profits taxes if they were held less than three years for immovable property, and, less than six months for movable property. Assets held longer than the specified periods were completely free from any tax.

The Finance Bill of 1965 introduced a long-term capital gains tax for individuals only. This applies to gains realized after April 6, 1965. The rate on long-term capital gains for individuals is a flat 30 per cent, but the taxpayer, at his option, may choose to include two-thirds of the gain in his ordinary income and have it subjected to the regular income tax and surtax.

Method of Payment

The British system of collection relies on the Pay-As-You-Earn system. The objective of this system is to collect the tax contemporaneously with the earning of the income so that, by the end of the year, the taxpayer will have paid, in most cases, exactly the amount owed to the Inland Revenue. The weekly deductions are adjusted to the condition of the taxpayer taking into account not only his income but also his exemptions. Each employee is given a code number by Inland Revenue representing his tax allowances, and the tax to be deducted is ascertained by the employer by reference to official tables.

The P.A.Y.E. system applies only to the income tax and not to the surtax. The tax obligations arising from the surtax are met in the year following the earning of the income.

III

A COMPARISON OF
THE INDIVIDUAL INCOME TAXES

There are basic differences among the various systems of individual income taxation[1]—in the treatment of the family, imputed rents, family allowances, interest, wages and salaries, capital gains, and dividends—that determine the productivity of the tax. However, the most important factor in determining the yield of the individual income tax is obviously per capita income. If two or more countries impose the same tax rates on the same "absolute" levels of income—assuming that the tax base is the same percentage of national income for each country, and that the income distribution is the same—the higher the per capita income of a country, the higher the ratio of the income tax revenue (T) to the national income (Y) will be. Likewise, the lower the per capita income of the country, the lower T/Y will be.[2]

What implication does this conclusion have in determining the subjective or psychological burden of the individual income tax? This is a very difficult question to answer since it involves interpersonal comparisons and value judgments about individuals. The comparison of large groups rather than individuals seems more justifiable.[3] Although one could defend intergroup comparisons in the same country (making some assumption of homogeneity about the population), it is hazardous to defend the same comparisons among different countries.

Suppose that there are two countries with comparable rates on equal (in an "absolute" sense) incomes. In both countries incomes of $5,000, given the same family situation, are taxed at the same rate of 20 per cent. If the per capita income in one country is $500 as opposed to $2,000 in the other, the taxpayer with an income of $5,000 might be in the highest decile of income

---

[1] See Chapter II for details with regard to each country.

[2] For a numerical example, see Communauté Economique Européenne, *Rapport du Comité Fiscal et Financier* (Brussels: 1962), p. 16. This study is commonly referred to as the *Neumark Report.*

[3] See Richard A. Musgrave, *The Theory of Public Finance* (New York: McGraw-Hill, 1959), p. 109.

distribution in the former and in the middle in the latter. In absolute terms the two taxpayers fare equally, but in relation to their position in society they do not, which may be crucial in determining their sense of well being.

If one adopts the relative measure of burden, then the same ratio of revenues from the personal income tax to national income (even for countries with quite different per capita incomes) presupposes the same burden. If an absolute measure of burden is used, the poorer country would have a much lower ratio of personal income tax to national income. How much lower the ratio ought to be depends on the difference in the per capita income of the two countries.

Casual theorizing and the implications of one of the theories of consumption[4] suggest that the relative position of an individual in the social setting in which he lives may be more important than the absolute level of income. The definition of a poor family in the United States as one with an income of less than $3,000 supports this position. In many other countries, a family with such an income would not be considered poor.

On the other hand, a case can be made that a certain tax percentage, on a given absolute income, will involve the same sacrifice—regardless of the per capita income of the country to which the taxpayer belongs—as long as the countries have "comparable civilizations." It has been maintained that France and the United States are two countries with "comparable civilizations" and that: "In France and in America we have the same notion of a standard diet, the same notion of lodging, the same notion of a minimum of comfort . . . all the progress of modern technics in the domain of the household are not in America, considered indispensable to the existence."[5]

The implication of this argument is carried to its extreme by other French authors who have maintained that the tax burden is the ratio of the revenue from the tax to the share of the national income which exceeds the subsistence income (*revenu national vital*). The absurdity to which this position is likely to lead is rather obvious, but a rejection does not invalidate the view that the absolute level of income must have something to do with the economic welfare of the individuals. If this were not true, we would not be so preoccupied with growth.

The truth is somewhere between the two extreme positions—i.e., comparison of tax rates at the same "absolute" level of income among countries, and comparison of taxes at the same "relative" level of income. I shall compare

[4]James S. Duesenberry, *Income, Saving and the Theory of Consumer Behavior* (Cambridge, Mass.: Harvard University Press, 1952).
[5]Maurice Lauré, "Impôts et Productivité," *Productivité Française*, No. 17, May 1953, p. 40 (my own translation).

the tax rates of the various countries according to each of these positions and let the reader draw his own welfare implications.[6]

ABSOLUTE INCOME METHOD

The first of these two methods of comparison, and the one which is commonly used, consists of specifying the family status of the taxpayer (i.e., single or married with one or more children), and of determining how much tax he would have to pay on given levels of income in each country.

A problem with this kind of comparison is that of rendering equivalent the incomes of different countries. One can express all incomes in the currency of one country (for example, in U.S. dollars) using the official rates of exchange. The disadvantage of this method is that the rates of exchange do not necessarily reflect the purchasing power of a given income in the various countries, and that the deviation of the purchasing power from the exchange rate is systematic being a function of the level of income in a country.[7] The second alternative is that of expressing all incomes in the currency of one country using cost of living rates of exchange. I give examples of both systems in my analysis.

Table III-1 provides estimates of the purchasing-power parities as percentages of exchange rates for the six countries. These estimates will be used in

[6]It should be fully realized, however, that, ceteris paribus, the same T/Y ratio for two countries implies that the poorer country is imposing higher tax rates on equal *absolute* income levels and that, vice versa, if two countries impose the same rates, the poorer country will show a lower T/Y. Strangely enough this fact does not seem to have been realized by many writers on the subject.

[7]Bela Balassa, "The Purchasing-Power Parity Doctrine: A Reappraisal," *Journal of Political Economy,* December 1964, pp. 584-96. Basing his case on several empirical studies, Balassa argues that the ratio of purchasing-power parities (calculated as a ratio of consumer goods prices for any pair of countries) to the exchange rate is an increasing function of income levels. This means, simply, that an income of, say, $2,000 will normally buy more goods and services in countries like Japan and Italy than in the United States. Thus, apart from the fact that such an income will be much higher in the percentile distribution of the former two countries than in the latter, it will be higher even in an absolute sense.

There is a further problem which should be at least mentioned. Even if one uses purchasing-power parities for reducing the incomes of different countries to the same common denominators, he would have succeeded in making equivalent only *average* incomes and not the income of each taxpayer regardless of his position on the income scale. In fact, the purchasing-power approach leaves much to be desired for our purpose insofar as it is unlikely that each taxpayer, regardless of the size of his income, buys the same composition of goods and services in the same proportion. For countries other than the United States, the purchasing-power approach would probably overstate the value, in terms of goods and services, of the high incomes and understate that of the low incomes; the opposite would be true for the United States. Conceptually this is a typical index number problem. For lack of information, however, this difficulty will be ignored and it will be assumed that no bias is created by the use of purchasing-power parities.

TABLE III-1. PURCHASING-POWER PARITIES AS PERCENTAGES OF
OFFICIAL EXCHANGE RATES, 1960

United States	100.0
United Kingdom	82.4
Germany	77.9
France	77.4
Italy	70.1
Japan	62.6

Source: Bela Balassa, "The Purchasing-Power Parity Doctrine: A Reappraisal," *Journal of Political Economy*, December 1964, p. 588. Balassa's data for the countries listed above are taken from I. B. Kravis and Michael W. S. Davenport, "The Political Arithmetic of International Burden-Sharing," *The Journal of Political Economy*, August 1963, pp. 327-29.

conjunction with the official rates to compare the personal income taxes of the various countries.[8]

Comparison of Personal Exemptions

Table III-2 gives the personal exemptions provided to single taxpayers and to families with two children. For single taxpayers—when the official rates of exchange are used—there is not much difference between the size of the exemptions allowed by the United States and the United Kingdom. On the other hand, those for Italy, Germany, and Japan are somewhat lower, while France does not allow a personal exemption. Putting the United States' exemption at 100, the United Kingdom's becomes 93, Germany's 70, Italy's 64, and Japan's 57. When married taxpayers with two dependent children are considered, the United States leads by a larger margin than for single taxpayers. In fact, no other country allows as much as 70 per cent of the United States' exemption.

Table III-2 also shows what happens to personal exemptions when, instead of using official rates of exchange, one uses purchasing-power parities. The British taxpayer now fares better than the single American taxpayer. Italian, Japanese, and German taxpayers are allowed exemptions which can buy only slightly less goods and services than their American counterpart.

For families with two children, however, the ranking is somewhat different. Here, the American family, in spite of the correction for the differences

[8]The data in Table III-1 are the most up-to-date of the various estimates available, but they refer to 1960 while the analysis for which they are being used centers around 1964. Since the cost of living did not increase equally in all of these countries, the actual purchasing-power parities for 1964—if they were available—would be somewhat different. What is more serious is that an analysis of the trends of the price indices of private consumption shows that the prices of the countries with the lowest purchasing-power parities in 1960 were the ones to increase fastest. In fact, curiously enough, there was a perfect but negative rank correlation between the data in Table III-1 and the rise in prices. This means that, if data for 1964 were available, the purchasing-power parities of all countries other than the U.S. and especially of those with a lower per capita income, would be a higher percentage than that of the U.S.

TABLE III-2. CHARACTERISTICS OF UPPER AND LOWER LEVELS OF
INDIVIDUAL INCOME TAX FOR SINGLE TAXPAYERS
AND FAMILIES WITH TWO CHILDREN

(in U.S. $ and percentages)

Country	Total personal exemption		First-bracket rate	Width of first bracket		Highest marginal rate	Income level at which it is reached	
	A	B		A	B		A	B
Single Taxpayer								
France	–	–	5%	$480 666[a]	$620 861[a]	65%	$14,400 20,000[a]	$18,604 25,800[a]
Germany	$420	$540	20	2,002	2,567	53[b]	27,500	35,260
Italy	384[c]	548[c]	4	1,152	1,643	80[d]	800,000	1,140,000
United Kingdom	560	672	20	280	340	91.25[f]	42,000	51,000
Japan	333	532	8	278	444	75	166,666	266,666
United States	600	600	14	500	500	70	100,000	100,000
Families with Two Children								
France	–	–	5	1,440 2,000[a]	1,860 2,600[a]	65	43,200 60,000[a]	55,812 78,000[a]
Germany	1,560	2,003	20	4,004	5,133	53[b]	55.000	70,538
Italy	624[c]	890[c]	4	1,152	1,643	80[d]	800,000	1,140,000
United Kingdom	1,610[e]	1,950[e]	20	280	340	91.25[f]	42,000	51,000
Japan	889[g]	1,422[g]	8	278	444	75	166,666	266,666
United States	2,400	2,400	14	1,000	1,000	70	200,000	200,000

Notes: A = at official rates of exchange.
  B = at cost of living (purchasing power) rates of exchange.

[a]For income from wages and salaries of which only 72 per cent is taxed. See Chapter II.

[b]Although the marginal incomes are taxed at this rate, some incomes just below the limits of the last column are taxed at 60 per cent. See Chapter II.

[c]Employment income. The exemption from the tax on the total income is much higher.

[d]This is the addition of the tax on incomes of category C_2, which reaches a maximum of 15 per cent (since 1965) on incomes over 20 million lire, and of the tax on total income which reaches a maximum of 65 per cent on incomes exceeding 500 million lire. For category A incomes, it could conceivably reach 92 per cent (or 96 per cent with other charges).

[e]Two children: one under eleven and the other between eleven and sixteen.

[f]This rate is the one in effect in 1965; in 1964 it was 88.75.

[g]Assumes that the income of the spouse is less than 50,000 yen and that the two children are one over and one under thirteen.

Sources: Chapter II and Table III-1.

in the cost of living of the various countries, is still ahead, but the lead has been substantially reduced.

Comparison of Statutory Rates

Comparisons of statutory rates are very difficult and require many assumptions concerning the ages of the children, the type of income taxed, the ages of the taxpayers, and other pertinent factors. Table III-2 shows some interesting aspects of the rate structure; for example, the size of the first-bracket rate is quite different from country to country. Generally, the countries which collect substantial revenues from the individual income taxes (the United States, Germany, and the United Kingdom) have relatively high first-bracket rates. Conversely those countries which collect low revenues (France, Italy, and, to a lesser extent, Japan) have lower first-bracket rates.

The effect of the different treatment of the family in each country is indicated in Table III-2. In this respect France is the most liberal, followed by the United States and Germany, both of which allow income splitting.[9] In the other three countries, the width of the bracket is the same, since they do not allow income splitting.

Additionally, Italy and France impose the lowest first-bracket rates on relatively wide first-brackets. This helps to explain the low revenues these two countries collect from this tax. Germany, on the other hand, imposes a very high first-bracket rate on a very wide bracket, which explains in part the substantial productivity of the German personal income tax, in spite of the absence of high progressivity.

The table also shows the maximum marginal rates and the levels of income at which they are reached. Of these the lowest is Germany's 53 per cent. The difference between this rate and the first rate is only 33 percentage points, which is why the German tax has usually been considered the least progressive of all. Furthermore, the income level at which the maximum rate is reached is relatively low. After Germany, there are three countries—France, the United States, and Japan—with approximately the same maximum rates.

The United Kingdom, with a marginal tax rate which reaches 90 per cent at relatively low incomes, imposes the heaviest taxes on high incomes. In Italy, however, the marginal rate would be applied to incomes of close to $1 million, which, whether they exist or not, do not appear in the declarations of the taxpayers. (There is no information published by the tax authority on the subject. From time to time, well-known personalities—often from the cinematographic industry—are reported by the Italian newspapers to have declared incomes so low as to make one wonder about the usefulness of having such high marginal rates on the books.)

[9]See Table III-4 for the effect that the French family quotients have on progressivity.

Table III-3 shows some comparative estimates of the average tax rates on given levels of incomes expressed in dollars (at official rates of exchange) for single individuals and for married couples with two children. "Taxable income" is income above the personal exemptions; the progressivity which is normally provided by these exemptions is therefore lost.

The table permits the following conclusions. For the low levels of income *above the personal exemptions*—say, up to $2,000—the United Kingdom and Germany impose the heaviest average rates. Germany may impose heavier rates on these income levels if the personal exemptions and the various other reliefs are taken into consideration. The United States imposes rates which are already substantial, while Japan, France, and especially Italy impose much lower rates. If the rates which had prevailed in the United States before the

TABLE III-3. AVERAGE INDIVIDUAL INCOME TAX RATES ON SELECTED
INCOMES FOR FAMILIES WITH TWO CHILDREN AND
FOR SINGLE TAXPAYERS, 1965

(percentages)

Taxable Income ($)	France S	France M	Germany S	Germany M	Italy[a]	United Kingdom 1964	United Kingdom 1965	Japan	United States S	United States M
280	0	0	20.0	20.0	0	20.0	20.0	n.a.	n.a.	n.a.
500	0	0	20.0	20.0	0	n.a.	n.a.	9.0	14.0	14.0
840	n.a.	n.a.	n.a.	n.a.	n.a.	26.6	26.6	n.a.	n.a.	n.a.
1,000	10.2	5.0	20.0	20.0	2.4	n.a.	n.a.	11.7	14.5	14.0
2,000	16.5	7.5	20.0	20.0	4.0	n.a.	n.a.	14.8	15.5	14.5
5,000	29.9	14.7	27.5	20.0	13.0	n.a.	n.a.	22.3	18.2	16.2
5,600	n.a.	n.a.	n.a.	n.a.	n.a.	36.9	39.0	n.a.	n.a.	n.a.
7,000	n.a.	n.a.	n.a.	n.a.	n.a.	39.3	41.5	n.a.	n.a.	n.a.
8,400	n.a.	n.a.	n.a.	n.a.	n.a.	41.3	43.5	n.a.	n.a.	n.a.
10,000	40.2	23.1	33.5	27.5	15.0	n.a.	n.a.	30.2	21.9	18.2
11,200	n.a.	n.a.	n.a.	n.a.	n.a.	45.0	47.3	n.a.	n.a.	n.a.
14,000	n.a.	n.a.	n.a.	n.a.	n.a.	48.3	50.6	n.a.	n.a.	n.a.
15,000	45.5	29.9	37.6	30.0	18.0	n.a.	n.a.	34.7	26.2	20.0
16,800	n.a.	n.a.	n.a.	n.a.	n.a.	51.3	53.6	n.a.	n.a.	n.a.
20,000	50.4	33.7	40.2	33.5	22.0	n.a.	n.a.	38.2	30.4	21.9
22,400	n.a.	n.a.	n.a.	n.a.	n.a.	56.3	58.9	n.a.	n.a.	n.a.
25,000	53.3	37.3	42.7	35.0	23.0	n.a.	n.a.	40.1	31.0	23.6
28,000	n.a.	n.a.	n.a.	n.a.	n.a.	60.3	62.7	n.a.	n.a.	n.a.
30,000	55.5	40.2	44.0	37.6	25.0	n.a.	n.a.	42.3	37.1	26.3
33,600	n.a.	n.a.	n.a.	n.a.	n.a.	63.4	66.2	n.a.	n.a.	n.a.
42,000	n.a.	n.a.	n.a.	n.a.	n.a.	68.3	70.7	n.a.	n.a.	n.a.
50,000	59.1	47.1	47.8	43.0	33.0	n.a.	n.a.	48.8	45.2	34.1
100,000	62.3	56.2	50.0	47.8	36.0	n.a.	n.a.	53.4	55.5	45.2
200,000	63.6	62.3	52.0	50.0	40.0	n.a.	n.a.	62.3	62.7	55.5

[a]Taxable Income for Italy includes the personal exemptions.

Sources: France: *Bulletin de Documentation Pratique des Impôts Directs et des Droits d'Enregistrement* (Paris: Editions F. Lefébvre, May 1966); Germany: *International Bureau of Fiscal Documentation, European Taxation* (Holland); Italy: *Stato dei Lavori della Commissione per lo Studio della Riforma Tributaria* (Milan: Giuffrè, 1964); United Kingdom: British Information Services, *The British System of Taxation* (1965); Japan: Ministry of Finance, *An Outline of Japanese Taxes* (Tokyo: yearly); United States: Richard Goode, *The Individual Income Tax* (Washington, D.C.: The Brookings Institution, 1964).

tax cut had been considered, the United States would have had rates similar to those of Germany and the United Kingdom.

For incomes of around $5,000, the United Kingdom again has the highest rates. Otherwise, bachelors in France and Germany are subjected to the heaviest taxes, while for families, Germany and Japan lead the way. The United States, France, and Italy are quite close together, with rates of around 15 per cent.

At income levels of $10,000 to $20,000, the taxes on the English families are still the heaviest, while those on French, German, and Japanese families are similar, leaving Italy and the United States with substantially lower rates. For bachelors the ranking is basically the same for all the countries, although the French are taxed at quite higher rates. The same ranking prevails at incomes of around $30,000, with the United Kingdom even further ahead of the others and with American and Italian families even further behind. For higher incomes (around $100,000), the United States catches up with Germany but is still behind France and Japan, with the United Kingdom at the head of the group and Italy at the end.

There is no doubt that the United Kingdom is the country with the highest rates on taxable income. These rates are so high that an income of $15,000, at the 1965 official rate of exchange, and about $18,000 at the cost of living rate of exchange, is reduced nearly 50 per cent by taxes. For the other countries, the 50 per cent average tax is not reached until the $100,000 income level.

TABLE III-4. EFFECT OF SPLITTING METHOD ON FRENCH AVERAGE
TAX RATES FOR SELECTED INCOMES, 1965

(percentages)

Taxable Income ($)	Family quotients			
	1	2	3	4
500	0	0	0	0
1,000	10.2	5.0	5.0	0
2,000	16.5	10.5	7.5	5.0
3,000	21.8	13.8	10.2	8.3
4,000	26.1	16.4	12.9	10.5
5,000	29.9	19.1	14.6	12.4

Source: Based on the 1965 Income Tax Law.

Italy has the lowest legal rates within the range of incomes considered. After Italy, the United States has the lowest rates for most incomes. For low incomes, however, the American rates are not low. In fact, for incomes of $2,000 and below, the United States rates are higher than those of France, Italy, and Japan. This is a reflection of the relatively high first-bracket rate and is certainly one of the main reasons for the high revenues from the

United States individual income tax. On the other hand, the French rate structure, with the combination of the splitting method and of low rates on low incomes, is such that low revenues are collected from this tax in spite of high rates on higher incomes. The effect of splitting on low income rates is shown in Table III-4. It should be recalled that the incomes in this table would be only 72 per cent in the case of wages and salaries.

RELATIVE INCOME METHOD

The above analysis suggests that the sacrifice an income tax imposes on an individual depends only on the absolute level of his income. But one could argue that two individuals have an equal tax sacrifice only when equal *relative* incomes are taxed equally. Furthermore, the nominal tax rates do not provide an estimate of the probable ratio of the revenue from the tax to the national income in each country. For example, suppose that a comparison of the nominal rates on taxable incomes of two countries shows that one of them treats low incomes favorably (especially if accompanied by high exemptions) and has very high rates for high incomes. The income tax burden will, nonetheless, be small, ceteris paribus, if the per capita income of this country is low. High tax rates on high incomes are important only for countries in which there are many large incomes. It is, therefore, necessary to account for differences in per capita incomes in making comparisons among different countries.

This can be done by expressing the income levels of each country as multiples of their per capita incomes, which could then be used to calculate the average income taxes. The implicit assumption here is that the income distributions of the various countries are basically identical. On the basis of this assumption a Frenchman with an income five times the French per capita income is in the same relative position as an American with an income five times the American per capita income.

Comparison of Personal Exemptions

Table III-5 compares the size of the personal exemptions for single taxpayers and married taxpayers with two children and the per capita income for each of the countries. Japan and Italy, two countries in which the revenues from the individual income tax are only a small share of the gross national product, have the highest percentage of personal exemptions for single taxpayers in relation to per capita income. The United States, on the other hand, provides a personal exemption that in relative terms is by far the smallest. This means that, ceteris paribus, the loss of taxable income due to the personal exemption is much lower in the United States than in the other countries. The United Kingdom provides a high personal exemption, which is quite significant in alleviating the weight of tax on low income groups.

TABLE III-5. RELATION BETWEEN PER CAPITA NATIONAL INCOME
AND PERSONAL EXEMPTIONS, 1963

(in national currencies and percentages)

Country	Per capita national income	Personal exemption	Personal exemption as a % of per capita national income	Total personal exemption for a family of four	Family exemption as a % of family income[a]
France[b]	6,234	-	-	-	-%
Germany	5,001	1,680	33.6	6,240	31.2
Italy[c]	436,000	240,000	55.1	390,000	22.4
United Kingdom	451	200	44.3	575	31.9
Japan	173,239	120,000	69.3	320,000	46.2
United States	2,526[d]	600[d]	23.7[d]	2,400[d]	23.7[d]
	2,850[e]	600[e]	21.1[e]	2,400[e]	21.1[e]

Notes: [a]Family income is assumed to be four times the per capita national income.

[b]France does not provide any personal exemption. However, an income which is below a certain minimum is not taxed. This minimum income is adjusted to the cost of living of the place of residence.

[c]Exemption applies to income from wages and salaries taxed with Schedule C_2 of *Ricchezza Mobile*.

[d]1965

[e]1963

Sources: For data on income: E.E.C., *General Statistical Bulletin* (Brussels); Great Britain, Central Statistical Office, *National Income and Expenditure* (London: H.M.S.O.); U.S., Council of Economic Advisers, *Economic Report of the President* (Washington, D.C.: G.P.O.); Japan, Economic Planning Agency, *Japanese Economic Statistics* (Tokyo). For other information, see Chapter II.

When families are considered, not much change is observed. The difference between the United States and the other countries decreases since in the United States each member of the family is allowed the same exemption, while, in the other countries, members other than the head of the family are allowed lower exemptions.

Comparison of Statutory Rates

Table III-6 shows the relative size of the bracket on which the first rate of the tax is applied. The countries where the individual income tax is less important (France, Italy, and Japan) impose a low rate on a relatively wide first bracket. Germany's first bracket is very wide, which explains why a large proportion of Germans are not taxed at progressive rates. The height of the first rate explains why the apparent lack of progressivity has not prevented the tax from providing substantial revenues.

The United Kingdom allows exemptions relatively higher than those of Germany. Once the income becomes taxable, it is immediately levied with a rate of about 20 per cent in both countries. While in Germany this rate

TABLE III-6. PERSONAL EXEMPTIONS AND LOWEST INCOME TAX BRACKETS,
AS PERCENTAGES OF PER CAPITA AND FAMILY INCOMES, 1963

(percentages)

Country	Single		Married with two children[a]		First-bracket tax rate
	Exemption	First bracket	Exemption	First bracket	
France	–	53.4[b]	–	40.1[b]	5
Germany	33.6	160.0	31.2	80.0	20[c]
Italy[d]	55.1	264.2	22.4	41.2	4
United Kingdom	44.3	22.2	31.9	5.5	20
Japan	69.3	57.8	46.2	14.4	8
United States	21.1[e]	17.3[e]	21.1[e]	8.7[e]	14[e]
	23.7[f]	79.2[f]	23.7[f]	39.6[f]	20[f]

Notes: [a]Family income is assumed to be four times the per capita income.
[b]Incomes from wages and salaries.
[c]The rate for 1965 is slightly lower.
[d]Incomes from wages and salaries (Schedule C_2, *Ricchezza Mobile*).
[e]1965.
[f]1963.

Sources: Same as Table III-5.

applies to incomes which are 1.6 times the per capita national income (or .8 the income of a standard family), in the United Kingdom it applies to incomes of only 22 per cent of the per capita income (or 5.5 per cent of the income of a standard family). Thus, the revenues the United Kingdom loses in the low incomes are recouped by taxes on high incomes.

In the United States, the tax cut of 1964 introduced greater progressivity in the low incomes by lowering the first rate and making it applicable to a smaller bracket. The most remarkable feature of the American tax is the very low personal exemption, which is probably one of the major reasons for the high productivity of the tax.

Table III-7 shows the average tax rates applicable to incomes expressed as multiples of the per capita national income of each country. This table is reproduced as Figure III-1 for the standard family and as Figure III-2 for the single taxpayer. Making the assumption that the distribution of income is basically the same in all six countries, the progression on relative incomes indicated by Table III-7 should help explain the differences in the tax burdens (T/Y) among the countries. The relative size of the exemptions and deductions (discussed on pp. 31-32) and differences in the erosion of the base of the individual income tax, which will be discussed in the following chapters, shed additional light on these differences.

TABLE III-7. AVERAGE INDIVIDUAL INCOME TAX RATES FOR
SINGLE TAXPAYERS AND MARRIED COUPLES WITH TWO CHILDREN
ON COMPARABLE RELATIVE INCOMES, 1965

(percentages)

Taxable income expressed as multiples of per capita incomes	France		Germany[a]		Italy	U.K.	Japan	United States	
	S	M	S	M				S	M
0.25	–	–	20.0	20.0	4.0	20.0	8.0	14.0	14.0
0.50	7.8	–	20.0	20.0	4.0	20.0	8.0	15.0	14.0
0.75	10.5	5.0	20.0	20.0	4.0	26.6	8.0	15.0	15.0
1.00	13.2	5.0	20.0	20.0	4.0	n.a.	9.0	16.0	15.0
1.50	16.8	7.8	21.1	20.0	4.0	n.a.	9.5	17.0	15.0
2.00	20.8	9.8	23.0	20.0	5.0	n.a.	11.0	19.0	16.0
3.00	27.0	13.2	25.0	21.1	5.0	n.a.	12.6	21.0	17.0
4.00	31.5	15.8	27.0	23.0	7.0	39.0	14.0	23.0	19.0
5.00	35.2	18.0	30.0	25.0	9.0	n.a.	16.0	26.0	20.0
10.00	44.4	28.8	36.0	27.0	10.0	45.0	22.0	37.0	26.0
20.00	54.5	39.2	43.0	36.0	18.0	56.0	31.2	45.0	37.0
30.00	57.9	44.4	n.a.	n.a.	20.0	68.0	35.0	55.0	45.0
100.00	n.a.	n.a.	n.a.	n.a.	31.0	n.a.	48.0	66.0	62.0

[a]The rates above are close approximations and refer to the 1958-64 period. The rates after 1964 were slightly lower.

Source: See Tables III-3 and III-5.

CONCLUSIONS

The analysis of the nominal rates in relation to the per capita income of each country leads to the following major conclusions.

The countries with a low ratio of the tax to the national income are (a) those for which the percentage of the personal exemption to the per capita income is the highest, and (b) those which impose a low first-bracket rate on a relatively wide first bracket. On the other hand, the countries with the highest ratio have lower personal exemptions and impose relatively high first-bracket rates on relatively wide first brackets.

The United States provides much smaller exemptions than the United Kingdom. The latter's relative exemptions are not only higher than those of the United States but they are also higher than those of Germany. This seems to be the main reason why the United States and Germany, with much lower nominal rates than the United Kingdom, have comparable revenues.

The United Kingdom imposes the highest relative rates on high incomes. Its tax structure is characterized by a relatively light treatment of low incomes and by a very heavy treatment of high incomes. In this respect it is different from Germany which levies heavy taxes on low incomes but relatively light taxes on high incomes.

The American tax is lighter than the German on incomes up to about ten times the per capita income. After that level it becomes heavier. The French

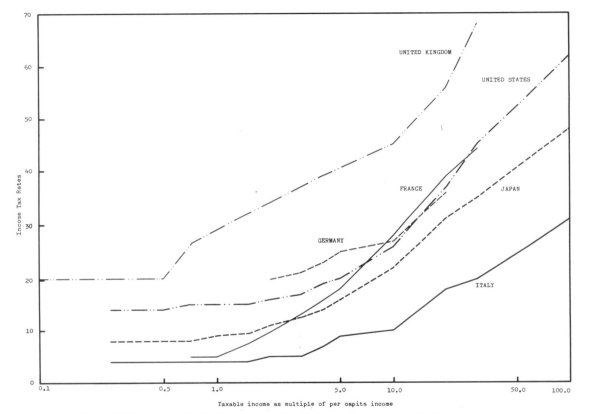

Figure III-1. Average Individual Income Tax Rates on Comparable Relative Incomes (Married Taxpayer with Two Children), 1965

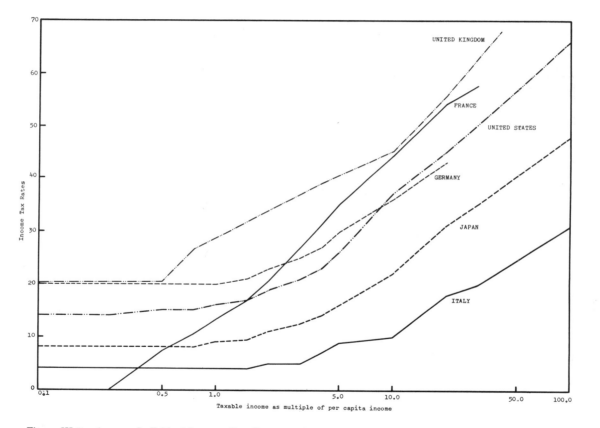

Figure III-2. Average Individual Income Tax Rates on Comparable Relative Incomes (Single Taxpayer), 1965

tax is heavy on single taxpayers, especially those with middle incomes; but the method of income splitting substantially alleviates the burden, especially for taxpayers in the high income brackets. Furthermore, there is evidence that tax evasion, especially at the high income levels, is more serious in France and Italy than in the other countries. Finally, at almost any relative income level, the nominal rates for Italy and Japan are lower than those for any of the other countries.

IV

INCOME TAX REVENUES AND PER CAPITA INCOME

Having considered the legal structures of the individual income taxes in the six countries, we turn now to actual revenues, which will be analyzed in relation to income brackets and then in the aggregate.

INCOME TAXES BY INCOME BRACKETS

France

The relevant data for France are given in Table IV-1 which provides a breakdown by the number of taxpayers, by income reported for taxation, and by the progressive income tax. Column (7) gives the average tax rate for each income bracket; this rate increases from around 5 per cent to around 50 per cent for high incomes (those above F500,000). In 1964 there were 7,725,028 taxpayers who reported combined incomes of over F96 billion (or F12,445 per return) and paid a little more than F12 billion (or about F1,555 per return).

The poorest 78 per cent of the taxpayers, with 51.63 per cent of the total reported income, paid only 34.34 per cent of the tax. The next 20.81 per cent with 38.73 per cent of reported income paid about 45 per cent of the tax. Finally, the top 1 per cent of the taxpayers, 79,477, with a combined income of 8.83 per cent of the total, paid 20.39 per cent of the tax.

There is evidence that the larger incomes claimed more family quotients. In fact, the average tax rate on families with many quotients was not lower than for those with few quotients. This is shown in Table IV-2.

Germany

Table IV-3 provides the most recent information available on the size distribution of the individual income tax in Germany by levels of income. Unfortunately, this table is limited to the wage and salary tax (*Lohnsteuer*) and thus it does not include the adjudicated, or assessed, income tax

TABLE IV-1. AVERAGE TAX RATE BY INCOME BRACKET
FOR FRANCE, 1964[a]

Income brackets in francs	Taxpayers		Total incomes		Progressive income tax		Average tax rate
	Thousands (1)	% (2)	million francs (3)	% (4)	million francs (5)	% (6)	(7)
10- 1,400	218	–	170	–	11	–	6.50
1,410- 2,500	44,563	0.58	92,614	0.10	4,676	0.03	5.05
2,510- 4,000	509,693	6.60	1,790,986	1.86	135,376	0.86	7.56
4,010- 6,500	1,541,398	19.95	8,100,832	8.43	801,632	5.01	9.90
6,510- 10,000	2,080,059	26.93	17,054,915	17.74	1,772,817	11.26	10.39
10,010- 15,000	1,854,493	24.01	22,596,516	23.50	2,705,153	17.18	11.97
15,010- 20,000	775,429	10.04	13,305,062	13.84	1,934,581	12.29	14.54
20,010- 36,000	663,737	8.59	17,008,193	17.01	3,186,177	20.23	18.73
36,010- 60,000	168,673	2.18	7,572,554	7.88	1,961,304	12.45	25.90
60,000-100,000	55,191	0.71	4,119,353	4.28	1,358,981	8.63	32.99
100,010-200,000	19,451	0.25	2,553,095	2.66	1,032,040	6.55	40.42
200,010-300,000	2,868	0.04	687,623	0.72	319,476	2.03	46.46
300,010-500,000	1,339	0.02	501,732	0.52	243,011	1.54	48.43
Over 500,000	628	0.01	624,789	0.65	257,710	1.64	41.25
Taxes calculated with particular rules	7,288	0.09	129,076	0.13			
Total	7,725,028	100.00	96,137,510	100.00	15,747,305	100.00	16.38
Net total					12,010,415		12.49

[a]On incomes of 1963.

Source: France, Ministère de l'Economie et des Finances, *Statistiques et Etudes Financières*, Supplement (Paris: Imprimerie Nationale, 18e année, Mai 1966.

TABLE IV-2. AVERAGE EFFECTIVE TAX RATE BY NUMBER OF
FAMILY QUOTIENTS FOR FRANCE, 1964

Family quotients	Rate	Family quotients	Rate
1	16.20	4	16.61
1.5	17.42	4.5	16.70
2	17.09	5	16.50
2.5	15.47	5.5	16.13
3	15.79	6	15.63
3.5	16.27	above 6	16.67

Source: Same as Table IV-1.

(*Einkommensteuer*) which normally is levied on incomes other than wages and salaries.

In 1961, there were 20,669,500 taxpayers who reported a combined gross income of about DM129 billion and paid over DM9 billion in tax. The income reported per taxpayer was DM6,230 and the tax paid was about DM450. The effective average tax rate increased from around 1 per cent on small incomes to 36.1 on incomes over DM100,000. The over-all average rate was 7.2 per cent.

The wage and salary tax seems to rely heavily on middle income groups. Thus, for example, the group between DM7,200 and DM20,000—about 31 per cent of the taxpayers and 52 per cent of the reported income—pays over 57 per cent of the tax. On the other hand, the top 1.12 per cent receives 5.45 per cent of the income and pays 13.33 per cent of the tax.

Italy

Data which make possible a classification of tax payments by level of income are not available for Italy. Italian published sources report incomes only by kind and not by level. This lack of data is not serious, however, because the amount of taxes paid by those with high incomes is probably so dismally low as to make it quite insignificant. In fact, the only progressive income tax which is imposed on high incomes is the *Imposta Complementare Progressiva.* Although, incomes classified under schedule A are probably associated with high incomes,[1] the fact remains that the only tax which tries to discriminate among incomes by level rather than by kind is the *Imposta Complementare.*

On paper, this is a very progressive tax with marginal rates reaching 65 per cent on incomes of over 500 million lire. According to the prevailing law, an

[1]The *Ricchezza Mobile* is imposed at 26 per cent on all income of category A. No exemption is allowed. Since these incomes were only 4.3 per cent of the taxed income, it follows that this was the percentage of taxed income hit by an average rate higher than 25 per cent.

TABLE IV-3. AVERAGE TAX RATE BY INCOME BRACKET FOR GERMANY, 1961

Income brackets in DM	Taxpayers		Total gross wages		Total wage tax		Average tax rate
	Thousands	%	Million DM	%	Million DM	%	
0- 2,400	3,531.0	17.08	4,210.3	3.26	31.7	0.34	0.75
2,400- 3,600	1,866.0	9.03	5,656.9	4.38	79.5	0.86	1.41
3,600- 4,800	2,437.0	11.79	10,291.7	7.98	381.1	4.11	3.70
4,800- 6,000	2,796.0	13.53	15,132.1	11.73	823.0	8.87	5.44
6,000- 7,200	2,968.0	14.36	19,587.9	15.18	1,077.2	11.60	5.50
7,200- 8,400	2,545.0	12.31	19,777.8	15.33	1,250.7	13.47	6.32
8,400- 9,600	1,646.4	7.97	14,742.5	11.43	1,026.4	11.06	6.96
9,600- 12,000	1,525.4	7.38	16,145.7	12.52	1,299.5	14.00	8.05
12,000- 16,000	835.8	4.04	11,393.4	8.83	1,154.0	12.43	10.13
16,000- 20,000	285.3	1.38	5,051.6	3.92	587.6	6.33	11.63
20,000- 25,000	131.7	0.64	2,903.6	2.25	377.8	4.07	13.01
25,000- 36,000	66.7	0.32	1,935.4	1.50	304.6	3.28	15.74
36,000- 50,000	21.1	0.10	873.0	0.68	171.2	1.84	19.61
50,000- 75,000	9.2	0.04	549.1	0.43	129.7	1.40	23.62
75,000-100,000	2.7	0.01	230.5	0.18	63.9	0.69	27.30
Over 100,000	3.1	0.01	526.0	0.41	190.1	2.05	36.10
Total	20,669.5	100.0	129,007.6	100.00	9,283.0	100.00	7.20

Source: Germany, Federal Office of Statistics, *Statistical Yearbook, 1966* (West Baden: 1966), p. 453.

income of 10 million lire is subjected to a tax of 11.63 per cent, and one of 100 million lire to a tax of 31.85 per cent. An income which does not exceed 960,000 lire is not subjected to the tax. Such an income is about twice the size of the per capita national income. This fact, together with the inevitable evasions, resulted in 1962 in only 2,909 billion lire or about 15 per cent of the national income being subjected to this tax. Furthermore, the average tax rate on this taxed income was only 3.3 per cent and the ratio of the tax to the national income was only .5 per cent. In other words, only .5 per cent of the national income of Italy was levied by progressive income taxation and most of this was levied with marginal rates not exceeding 10 per cent.

United Kingdom

The relevant data for the United Kingdom is provided in Table IV-4. There were 27.5 million taxpayers in 1964; they reported an aggregate income of £22,885 million (£832 per return) and paid £2,617 million (£95 per return). The average tax rate by income bracket goes up to 74.36 per cent, while the over-all average rate is 11.44.

It is obvious that this tax is very heavy on the high income brackets: the top 405,000 taxpayers, (or 1.46 per cent of the total), who received 10.04 per cent of the income, paid 33.36 per cent of the tax. On the other hand, to get an equivalent amount of tax from the low income brackets, the Inland Revenue had to tax about 10 million people. The bottom 36 per cent of the

TABLE IV-4. AVERAGE TAX RATE BY INCOME BRACKET
FOR THE UNITED KINGDOM, 1964

Income brackets in £	Taxpayers		Total reported income		Total income tax and surtax		Average tax rate
	Thousands	%	Million £	%	Million £	%	
50- 250	3,985	14.49	770	3.36	–	–	–
250- 300	1,590	5.78	434	1.90	–	–	–
300- 400	2,280	8.29	806	3.52	11	0.42	1.36
400- 500	2,115	7.69	951	4.16	33	1.26	3.47
500- 600	1,970	7.16	1,083	4.73	53	2.03	4.89
600- 700	1,940	7.05	1,260	5.51	75	2.87	5.95
700- 800	1,920	6.98	1,440	6.29	94	3.59	6.53
800- 1,000	3,765	13.69	3,374	14.74	239	9.13	7.08
1,000- 1,500	5,485	19.95	6,583	28.77	600	22.93	9.11
1,500- 2,000	1,450	5.27	2,475	10.81	350	13.37	14.14
2,000- 3,000	595	2.16	1,412	6.17	289	11.04	20.47
3,000- 5,000	254	0.92	957	4.18	259	9.90	27.06
5,000-10,000	119	0.43	800	3.50	288	11.00	36.00
10,000-20,000	26	0.09	345	1.51	181	6.92	52.46
20,000 and over	6	0.02	195	0.85	145	5.54	74.36
Total	27,500	100.00	22,885	100.00	2,617	100.00	11.44

Source: Great Britain, Central Statistical Office, *National Income and Expenditure, 1966* (London: H.M.S.O.).

taxpayers, receiving about 13 per cent of the income, paid only 1.68 per cent of the total tax. Finally, 91.11 per cent of the taxpayers, with a combined income of 73 per cent of the total, paid only 42.23 per cent of the tax. The average effective tax rate for the highest bracket within this group (£1,000–£1,500) was only 9.11 per cent.

Japan

Table IV-5 gives the data on the distribution of the Japanese individual income tax by income brackets for 1963. Over 10 million taxpayers reported a combined income of 10,214 billion yen (about $28 billion) and paid 5.6 per cent of this income in taxes. The average taxpayer reported an income of 535 thousand yen ($1,485) and paid a tax of 30,055 yen (about $84).

The average effective tax rate by income brackets increases from 1 to over 40 per cent; however, the number of taxpayers (and the percentage of reported income) hit by high rates is really very small. Only 1,000 taxpayers were taxed with average rates of over 40 per cent, and only 38,000 with average rates above 20 per cent. The percentage of reported income taxed with average rates above 20 per cent was about 3 per cent. For 98 per cent of the taxpayers—or 90 per cent of the income—the average effective rate remained below 10 per cent. Thus, it is obvious that for most Japanese the individual income tax was not much heavier than most of the sales taxes. Because of the very low tax payments of low and middle incomes and because of the low over-all average rate, the share of the tax paid by the taxpayers who reported high incomes was quite substantial: The top 2 per cent paid 33.5 per cent of the tax, and the top 8 per cent paid 58.8 per cent.

TABLE IV-5. AVERAGE TAX RATE BY INCOME BRACKET
FOR JAPAN, 1963

Income brackets in yen (thousands)	Taxpayers		Total reported income		Total tax		Average tax rate
	Thousands	%	Million yen	%	Million yen	%	
0- 200	2,087	10.9	368,777	3.6	3,800	0.7	1.0
200- 300	3,724	19.5	935,373	9.2	20,261	3.5	2.2
300- 500	6,022	31.6	2,399,819	23.5	58,637	10.2	2.4
500- 700	3,688	19.3	2,151,704	21.1	66,165	11.5	3.1
700- 1,000	2,031	10.6	1,654,579	16.2	87,819	15.3	5.3
1,000- 2,000	1,215	6.4	1,585,361	15.5	144,885	25.3	9.1
2,000- 5,000	277	1.5	800,652	7.8	113,923	19.8	14.2
5,000-10,000	32	0.2	209,779	2.0	42,336	7.4	20.2
10,000-20,000	5	0.0	66,848	0.7	19,480	3.4	29.1
Over 20,000	1	0.0	41,558	0.4	16,738	2.9	40.3
Total	19,082	100.0	10,214,450	100.0	574,044	100.0	5.6

Source: Japan, Ministry of Finance, Tax Bureau, *Major Statistics of Taxation in Japan* (Tokyo, 1965). [available only in Japanese]

However, even though the distribution of the tax was uneven, the average rates were so low that it is unlikely that the savings of the high income groups could have been affected in a significant fashion. Thus, for example, the 58.8 per cent of the tax levied from the top 8 per cent was taxed with an average rate of only 12.5 per cent.

Conclusions

To draw some conslusions from the data of this section, I have made use of Lorenz curves (Figure IV-1) to relate the destribution of reported income to that of the tax paid for all the countries except Italy. These curves make it possible to compare the evenness of the tax distribution in relation to taxed income.[2]

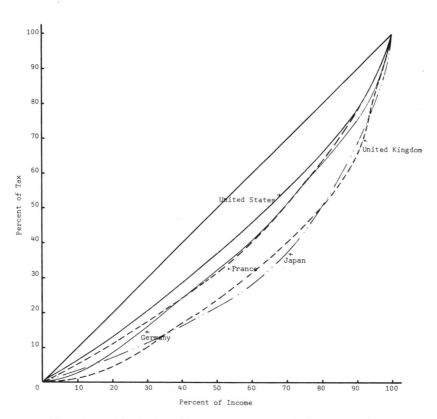

Figure IV-1. Distribution of Income Tax Revenues by Income Bracket

[2]The Lorenz curves could have been used in relation to taxpayers rather than taxed income.

Some aspects of these curves are of particular importance. The United States, and this comes as a surprise, has the most even distribution of the tax among the income brackets. The United Kingdom has the most uneven distribution. In the United Kingdom, the low income brackets (up to about 40 per cent of the total reported income) contribute the smallest share of any country to the total tax while the top 20 per cent of income contributes more to the total tax in the United Kingdom than anywhere else.

The lowest 30 per cent of the income contributes about 10 per cent of the tax in the United Kingdom, about 12 per cent in Japan, about 16 per cent in Germany, 18 per cent in France, and over 20 per cent in the United States. At the other extreme, the top 10 per cent contributes about 35 per cent in the United Kingdom, 30 per cent in Japan, 22 per cent in Germany, and about 20 per cent in the United States and France.

ALTERNATIVE MEASURES OF NATIONAL INDIVIDUAL INCOME TAX BURDENS

In the previous section I have analyzed the revenues from the individual income tax by income brackets. Here I shall deal with these revenues from the point of view of a whole country rather than specific income groups.

Table IV-6 provides three different ways of looking at the burden of the individual income tax in each country. The first column gives the most common definition. In 1963 the United States was the country with the

TABLE IV-6. ALTERNATIVE DEFINITIONS OF INCOME TAX BURDENS
FOR SIX COUNTRIES, 1963

(percentages and U.S. $)

Country	IT/PI	$\bar{Y}_e$	Index of $\bar{Y}_e$	$\dfrac{IT/PI}{\bar{Y}_e \text{ index}}$	$\bar{Y}_p$	Index of $\bar{Y}_p$	$\dfrac{IT/PI}{\bar{Y}_p \text{ index}}$
United States	10.2%	$2,454	100.0%	10.2%	$2,454	100.0%	10.2%
France	3.1	1,342	54.7	5.7	1,734	70.7	4.4
Germany	9.0	1,324	54.0	16.7	1,700	69.3	13.0
Italy	4.2	702	28.6	14.7	1,002	40.8	10.3
United Kingdom	9.9	1,318	53.7	18.4	1,600	65.2	15,2
Japan	4.2	458	18.7	22.5	732	29.8	14.1

Notes: $\bar{Y}_e$ = Per capita GNP in U.S. $ at official rates of exchange.

$\bar{Y}_p$ = Per capita GNP in U.S. $ at purchasing-power parities.

Sources: Table III-1; U.S., Council of Economic Advisers, *Economic Report of the President* (Washington, D.C.: G.P.O., annual); France, Ministère des Finances, *Statistiques et Etudes Financières* (Paris: monthly); Germany, Deutsche Bundesbank, *Monthly Report* (Frankfurt Am Main: monthly); Italy, Ministero delle Finanze, *L'Attività Tributaria dal 1954 al 1964* (Rome: Istituto Poligrafico dello Stato, 1965); Japan, Ministry of Finance, Tax Bureau, *An Outline of Japanese Taxes* (Tokyo: annual); Great Britain, Central Statistical Office, *National Income and Expenditure* (London: H.M.S.O., annual); E.E.C., General Statistical Bulletin (Brussels: monthly).

highest income tax burden, followed by the United Kingdom and Germany. These three countries had ratios of around 10 per cent, while France, Italy, and Japan had ratios of around 4 per cent.[3]

The fourth column provides an alternative definition of individual income tax burden which takes into consideration the per capita income of the country. It is obtained by dividing the figures in the first column by an index of the per capita personal income of each country. This is an adaptation of a method for measuring the total tax burden of different countries (or different states) suggested recently.[4] The results obtained by its use are strikingly different from those obtained by the previous method. In fact, now the United States appears to be a country with a relatively light individual income tax burden; only France seems to have a lighter burden. Japan and the United Kingdom with burdens of 22.5 and 18.4 respectively are ahead of the other countries. The most remarkable shift is that of Japan from 4.2 to 22.5 while Germany moves from 9 to 16.7. A variance of this method is obtained in the last three columns of the table by using purchasing-power rates of exchange. The effect of this change is to decrease the burdens of all the countries other than that of the United States and thus bring them closer to the burdens in the first column. The United Kingdom is now ahead of any other country— with a burden of 15.2—and Japan follows; Germany still leads the United States by about 3 percentage points. Italy's burden is just about that of the United States while France's falls back.

These three alternative measures of the income tax burdens show how difficult it is to have an objective criterion for making these comparisons. An attempt at suggesting such a criterion is made in the following section.

A NEW METHOD FOR COMPARING THE BURDENS OF THE INCOME TAX

So far the problem of comparison of income tax burdens has been approached from two viewpoints: a comparison of nominal rates, and of the ratios of the revenues from the income tax to personal income.

It is obvious that these two methods give significantly divergent results whenever the per capita incomes of the countries are substantially different. For example, if two or more countries impose the same tax rates on the same levels of income, and if (a) the base of the income tax is the same ratio of the national income for each country, (b) the degree of tax evasion does not differ from country to country, and (c) the income distributions are identical, then, the higher the per capita income of a country is, the higher the ratio of

[3]If the denominator had been GNP, the United Kingdom would have shown the highest ratio.

[4]Richard Bird, "A Note on Tax Sacrifice Comparison," *National Tax Journal,* September 1964, pp. 303-8.

the income tax revenue to the national income will be. Mutatis mutandis the same ratio for two or more countries implies that the poorer country is imposing higher tax rates on given income levels and that, vice versa, if two countries impose the same rates, the poorer country will show a lower ratio.

Thus, the simple comparison of ratios of revenues to national incomes does not reveal much about the level of the effective tax rates. On the other hand, a comparison of nominal rates on taxable income is never conclusive since it abstracts from problems of evasion, erosion of tax base, etc., and, furthermore, it is always limited to typical taxpayers such as bachelors, married couples with a certain number of children, and so forth. The results obtained from comparing this typical taxpayers cannot be generalized to the whole countries.

In view of the limitations of these two approaches and of their often conflicting results, and in view of the fact that the base of the income tax and the degree of evasion are different from country to country, it would be useful to have a less ambiguous method for the comparison that would implicitly take into account not only the differences in per capita incomes but also the different degrees of erosion of the income tax bases and the different degrees of evasion in the various countries. One possibility would be a method that would attempt to answer the following question: Assume that the U.S. federal income tax laws were being applied not only in the United States but also in the other countries, how would the resulting ratios of the revenues from this tax to the personal incomes for these countries compare with the ratios that they obtain from the application of their own income tax laws?

Description of the Method[5]

The method suggested here is based on the fact that the federal individual income tax in the United States is collected from fifty states which have widely different per capita incomes, and that the same set of tax rules and rates that applies, for example, in Nevada and Delaware which in 1963 were the states with the highest per capita incomes, applies also in South Carolina and Mississippi, those with the lowest.

If one or several states could be located with approximately the same per capita income as the foreign country with which one wishes to compare the United States, one could simply calculate the ratio of this tax to the personal income of that state (or states) and compare this ratio with the one that the foreign country gets from its own income tax. This would be a rudimentary but direct way of telling what the American income tax would yield if

[5] An elaboration of the following discussion will be found in my article, "Comparing International Tax Burdens: A Suggested Method," *Journal of Political Economy,* October 1968.

applied to the foreign country and if the foreign country had the same
characteristics as the American state. It would, however, suffer from the
anomalies of particular states.

The method can be refined by a simple application of regression analysis.
In fact, by taking the individual income tax burden by state and regressing it
against the per capita personal income also by state, a regression equation is
obtained that indicates an estimated relationship between various levels of
income and the corresponding tax burden, *given the American Federal
income tax*. Or, $\frac{T_i}{Y_i} = f(\overline{Y}_i)$, where $i = 1 \ldots 50$, and T_i, Y_i, and $\overline{Y}_i$ are respectively the total income tax revenue, total personal income, and per capita
personal income for the state i.

The data used for the estimation of the desired relationship are readily
available.[6] From them it can be seen that the ratio of the income tax revenue
to the personal income is obviously a function of the per capita income of
each state. In fact, that ratio goes from a low of 6.8 for Mississippi to over 12
for Nevada, Delaware, and Connecticut which in 1963 were the three states
with the highest per capita personal income.

The regression equation is:

$$\frac{T_i}{Y_i} = 3.91 \ + 0.00253 \ \overline{Y}_i$$

$$(0.00020) \qquad\qquad\qquad r^2 = 0.77$$

The equation indicates that when the American federal income tax is
applied a \$400 change in per capita income is associated with about a 1 per
cent change in the ratio of revenue to income. Therefore, by substituting for
$\overline{Y}_i$ the per capita income of the foreign countries with which one wants to
compare the burden of the American income tax, it is possible to get an
estimate of the most likely burdens that these countries would have if their
personal incomes were being levied with a tax which had the same rates and
the same characteristics as the American federal income tax and which was
being levied with the same rules and the same degree of enforcement as in
the United States. In other words one would get the most likely burdens that
these foreign countries would get if they were American states.

The application of the method shows that while the estimated burdens for
the fifty American states go from 7.4 to 12.5, those for the five foreign
countries go from 5.8 to 8.3. Comparing the actual with the estimated

[6]U.S., Department of Commerce, *Statistical Abstract of the United States*
(Washington, D.C.: G.P.O., 1966); U.S., Internal Revenue Service, *Statistics of Income*
(Washington, D.C.: G.P.O., 1966).

burdens for the foreign countries, it becomes clear that the actual income tax burdens of France, Italy, and Japan are much lower than what they would be if they were American states and, thus, were subjected to the federal income tax; if they were American states, or if the effective rates of their income taxes were as heavy as the American, the French burden would have been 2.68, the Italian 1.52, and the Japanese 1.38 times higher. Statistically the differences between their estimated and their actual ratios are significant at the 1 per cent level.

On the other hand the imposition of the American income tax would have probably lowered the British and the German burden. In fact, the British actual burden was 1.24 times what it would be expected to be from the regression line, and the German's was 1.1 times higher. However, while this difference is statistically significant at the 1 per cent level for the United Kingdom, it is not significant for Germany.

In conclusion, the results obtained show that, in 1963, of the six countries considered, the United Kingdom had the heaviest personal income tax followed respectively by Germany, the United States, Japan, Italy, and France. The application of this method thus shifts the rank of the United States from the first to the third place and implies that the American income tax is not as heavy as it is normally believed.

V

INCOME TAX TREATMENT OF
DIFFERENT KINDS OF INCOME

This chapter provides a comparative analysis of the methods of taxation employed vis-à-vis different kinds of income. The income tax treatment of wages and salaries will be compared with that of other incomes. Whenever feasible the other incomes have been broken down into major categories.

There are three reasons for this kind of analysis. The first has to do with the different marginal propensity to save out of different kinds of income. It has been assumed, at least since the times of Ricardo, that the marginal propensity to save out of wages and salaries is somewhat lower than that of other incomes. This assumption has received substantial empirical backing recently.[1] Thus, it is important to know the relative share of revenues from individual income tax which each major income category is contributing in order to assess the impact that this tax may have had on personal saving. The second concerns the "propensity to evade" the tax, which also depends on the kind of income that is being levied since some incomes can be controlled more easily than others. Finally, it is interesting to know how the industrial countries have effectively discriminated in their treatment of different incomes since this discrimination, if intentional, is a reflection of their attitude toward equity and growth.

INDUSTRIAL AND FUNCTIONAL DISTRIBUTION
OF NATIONAL INCOME

Agriculture has traditionally proved to be rather refractory to income taxation. Table V-1 gives the share of national income originating in this sector. Without attempting to attribute causality, it is worth noting that there is a strong negative rank correlation between the importance of agriculture in the economy and the importance of income as a basis of taxation. Conversely, it would seem that the industrialization of a country facilitates the

[1]H. S. Houthakker, "An International Comparison of Personal Savings," *International Statistical Bulletin* (Tokyo), May-June 1960; Nicholas Kaldor, "Alternative Theories of Distribution," *Review of Economic Studies,* No. 62, 1955-56.

TABLE V-1. SHARE OF AGRICULTURE, FORESTRY, AND FISHING IN THE
DOMESTIC PRODUCTS OF SIX COUNTRIES, SELECTED YEARS

(percentages)

Years	France[a,b]	Germany[b]	Italy[b]	U.K.[b,c]	U.S.[d]	Japan[d]
1955	11.4	8.0	23.2	4.8	4.5	23.0
1958	10.6	7.1	20.1	4.3	4.7	18.5
1961	8.8	5.5	17.7	4.0	4.0	14.4
1964	7.8	4.8	14.7	3.6	3.3	12.7

[a]Excludes fishing, includes the production of wine.

[b]Gross domestic product.

[c]Includes stock appreciation.

[d]Net domestic product.

Source: O.E.C.D., *National Accounts Statistics, Expenditure, Product and Income, 1955-1964* (Paris: O.E.C.D., 1966).

imposition of income taxes. If the industrial outputs of the six countries were taken as percentages of their gross national products, a strong positive rank correlation between those percentages and the countries' reliance on income taxation would result. The reason for this is rather obvious: With a decrease in the importance of agriculture and an increase in that of industry, the share of national income which is obtained from dependent work (mainly wages and salaries) increases, while income is at the same time generated in fewer economic units; thus, it becomes easier to check on the income of people and to use it as a basis for taxation. Therefore, the share of wages and salaries in the national income should also be of interest. This is given in Table V-2.

Income taxes on wages and salaries cannot be evaded, or at least it is much harder to do so, which provides a good ground for a lighter treatment of these

TABLE V-2. SHARE OF WAGES AND SALARIES IN THE NATIONAL INCOME
OF SIX COUNTRIES

(percentages)

Years	France	Germany	Italy	Japan	U.K.	U.S.
1955	57.5	58.8	50.8	48.5	72.6	67.6
1956	58.0	59.5	51.8	48.7	72.8	69.1
1957	58.6	59.7	51.8	49.1	72.6	69.7
1958	58.3	60.5	51.9	52.2	72.3	69.9
1959	59.5	60.2	51.7	50.9	71.8	69.5
1960	58.3	60.8	52.1	50.0	72.5	70.7
1961	60.5	62.5	52.3	50.2	73.3	70.5
1962	60.7	64.0	54.6	52.7	74.1	70.5
1963	62.9	64.7	58.7	53.5	73.1	70.6
1964	64.1	64.7	59.9	54.8	73.8	70.8
1965	64.8	66.0	59.7	55.6	73.9	70.0

Source: O.E.C.D., *National Accounts Statistics, 1955-1964* (Paris: O.E.C.D., 1966); and O.E.C.D., *National Accounts Statistics, 1956-1965* (Paris: O.E.C.D., 1967).

incomes. In fact, if they are treated in the same way as other incomes, and if the assumption is true that taxes on them are difficult to evade, then a de jure nondiscriminatory treatment of these incomes would amount to a de facto discrimination. Because of this, most countries have granted some favorable treatment to these incomes, which have ranged from the simple discrimination implied in the schedular tax system of Italy to the more subtle discrimination used in France and the United Kingdom. The only country of those considered which does not provide special treatment for these incomes is the United States.

TAX TREATMENT OF WAGES AND SALARIES

In Italy, incomes from wages and salaries are taxed according to schedule C_2, the lightest of all the schedules used in 1965, which had a range in rates of 4 to 15 per cent.[2] However, even at 1965 rates, it is very unlikely that many people have to pay more than 10 per cent on this kind of income since this average rate applies to incomes from wages and salaries of 10 million lire (approximately twenty times the per capita income of the country).[3] In relative terms, this would correspond in the United States to an income from this source of over $50,000. Salaries of this relative size are not too common even in the United States in spite of the large number of professional managers in industries. In Italy, where there are fewer professional managers, the number of very high incomes from dependent work is more limited.

France does not have a schedular system. However, only 72 per cent of incomes from wages and salaries are taxable, with a further reduction of 5 per cent after the tax has been calculated.[4] Furthermore, with the increase in importance of transfer payments, which are deductible, the share of income from work which remains taxable is smaller. This is also true for Italy and Germany.

In Germany the law allows a standard deduction of DM564 from wages and salaries in order to cover the expenses connected with employment. If the expenses are itemized and exceed DM564 a further deduction is allowed. Incomes from capital give rise also to a deduction, but for these the deduction is only DM150.

The United Kingdom provides important deductions for "earned" income, but it taxes family allowances, although some other kinds of transfer pay-

[2] The maximum was raised from 8 per cent in 1964.

[3] Actually if the tax on the schedule C_2 of *Ricchezza Mobile* and the *Imposta Complementare* are added together, the average tax rate at this level may be around 18 per cent; it would be somewhat higher for other incomes.

[4] See Chapter II.

ments are tax exempt. It is restrictive in its treatment of expenses connected with employment which must be "wholly, exclusively and necessarily incurred." Furthermore, for the United Kingdom, "earned" income does not mean in the strictest sense income from work (which includes professional income) but also mixed income. The latter requires the cooperation of labor and capital. Thus, the incomes which are not "earned" are exclusively incomes from personal investments (dividends, interest, etc.). The latter are the incomes which are hit most by the surtax.[5] In short, rather than discriminating in favor of income from "dependent" work, England discriminates against income from personal investments.

Japan also provides some preferential treatment for employment income. The taxpayer is allowed the following deductions: if the income received does not exceed 410,000 yen, he may deduct 20,000 yen plus 20 per cent of the income over 20,000 yen; for incomes between 420,000 and 820,000 yen, he may deduct 100,000 yen plus 10 per cent of the excess over 420,000 yen. For incomes exceeding 820,000 yen, he may deduct 140,000 yen.

In the United States, there is no favorable treatment of wages and salaries as such.

REASONS FOR FAVORABLE TREATMENT OF INCOME FROM WORK

Cost of Earning Income

Discrimination in favor of income from work can and has been defended for other reasons besides the possibility of evasion. There have been many public finance discussions which have defended such differential treatment on the ground that to earn income from work requires a greater cost than to earn an equivalent income from invested capital. The taxpayer is only partially compensated for the cost of earning his living by the permissible deduction of tools, uniforms, and other expenses. For example, the taxpayer is not compensated in the United States under the standard deduction. Furthermore, there are always other expenses (such as transportation costs in terms of both time and money) which are normally not deductible. Besides, income from work is always of a temporary nature; there is, therefore, the need to provide for the future through saving. In this case it seems reasonable that saving from employment income should be exempted. This is one of the arguments used in favor of an expenditure tax.[6]

[5]See pp. 70-71 for statistical information.

[6]Nicholas Kaldor, *An Expenditure Tax* (London: George Allen & Unwin Ltd., 1965); Luigi Einaudi, *Saggi sul Risparmio e l'Imposta* (Torino: Giulio Einaudi Editore, 1958).

Evasion

It has been argued that because administration of the Italian income tax is inefficient a schedular income tax is more equitable[7] and that the real progressivity of the Italian income tax is owing mainly to its schedular character; given a good tax administration, there would be no need for a schedular tax system.[8] But, given the actual administration, the schedular system provides some progressivity to the income tax which would be lacking without the discrimination in favor of wages and salaries. This is probably right, but it amounts to a legalization of evasion and inevitably hurts the honest taxpayers. The Commissione per lo Studio della Riforma Tributaria has argued against the schedular system for the following reason: "In order to avoid [tax] evasion no remedy is possible but an effort aimed at preventing it; it is not justifiable to legalize it with [different rates]."[9]

Methods of Collection

Differential treatment of the various kinds of income may also be a consequence of the way in which income taxes are collected. Discrimination of this kind is not intentional but it does exist. Taxes on income can either be collected at the source or they can be paid at a specified future date, normally in the following year. If they are collected at a future date, if the country's per capita income is growing, and if the ratio of the tax to the income on which it is calculated remains the same, then the real tax burden— i.e., the ratio of the tax payment at the time the tax is paid to the income of that same period—will be lower.[10] Formally, define T_t as the tax calculated on an income Y_t, and assume that $T_t = aY_t$. Now, if the ratio $\dfrac{T_t}{Y_t} = a$ is a constant, and if the tax T_t is collected in a later period $t+1$ when, due to growth, $Y_{t+1} > Y_t$, then the real tax burden will be $T_t = bY_{t+1}$ or $\dfrac{T_t}{Y_{t+1}}$ so that $a > b$.

---

[7]Francesco Forte, "Comment on Schedular and Global Income Taxes," *Readings on Taxation in Developing Countries,* ed. Richard Bird and Oliver Oldman (Baltimore: The Johns Hopkins Press, 1964), pp. 185-86. Professor Harberger has used the same argument to suggest that in Latin America income from capital be taxed at higher rates than income from dependent work. See Arnold G. Harberger, "Issues of Tax Reform for Latin America," Organization of American States, *Fiscal Policy for Economic Growth in Latin America* (Baltimore: The Johns Hopkins Press, 1965), pp. 110-20.

[8]*Ibid.*

[9]Commissione per lo Studio della Riforma Tributaria, *Stato dei Lavori della Commissione per lo Studio della Riforma Tributaria* (Milan: Giuffré, 1964), p. 165.

[10]See J. Parent, "Impôt Progressif, Matière Fiscale et Croissance Economique," *Revue de Science Financière,* No. 3, 1956.

By how much a will exceed b will depend, ceteris paribus, on the rate of growth of the country at current prices. If the national income is growing at a rate of 3 per cent per year, and if $a = .1$ or 10 per cent, then b will be 9.7 per cent. If the rate of growth is 5 per cent, b will be 9.5 per cent. Of course, if the country is growing at an accelerating pace, the real charge of the income tax will be decreasing. This will be particularly true in periods of inflation which will reduce the "real" value of tax payments.

How important this effect will be for a country depends on the method of collection, the length of the lag between the time the income is earned and the time the tax is paid, the rate of growth of the country, the rate of inflation, and the importance of the income tax in the fiscal system of the country. Thus if the national income of a country is $100 billion and the tax on that income is $10 billion or 10 per cent and is paid in the following period when the income has grown, say, to $110, then, the actual burden of the tax will be about 9 per cent, or, about $1 billion less. Therefore, the impact of the income tax on consumption and saving will be less than expected from the nominal rates if the lag in payment is ignored.

This issue is mentioned since Germany, the United Kingdom, the United States, Japan, and, to a lesser extent, Italy withhold at the source a substantial part of the taxes on income from wages and salaries; thus the tax is paid approximately at the same time the income is earned. In the United Kingdom and Germany, most of the other taxes on incomes, other than those on wages and salaries, are normally paid some time later.

In the United Kingdom, the Pay-As-You-Earn system has carried withholding of taxes further than in any other country. This system attempts to approximate as closely as possible the tax currently owed by the taxpayer in order for him not to have to make any payment at the end of the fiscal year. This is true only of the income tax and not of the surtax. Payments for the surtax are not due until about a year after the income has been earned. Since the surtax is largely a tax on income from investments (dividends, interest, etc.), it is clear that the differential treatment compensates for the reliefs provided to earned income.

The net effect of this system can be visualized in two ways. First, one can say that some forms of income are given an interest free loan, so that the net saving to these incomes is equivalent to the interest rate which the tax liability can earn from the time the income is earned until the tax is paid. Alternatively, the actual (or real) rate of taxation on incomes subject to the surtax is obtained by dividing the tax payment at a certain period by the tax base in that same period rather than in the period when the income was earned.

Germany's taxes on wages are also usually withheld at the source and thus their payment is simultaneous with the earning. The same is true for the tax on capital returns (*Kapitalertrag*). The story is different for the adjudicated (*Veranlagte*) taxes, which are set by the field officers on the basis of information submitted by the taxpayer. It takes from one to three years before final payments are made. In the meantime people submit quarterly payments on the basis of the income of the previous period. In a growing economy, this will amount to a tax free loan.

In the United States this also holds true to a limited extent since the law requires that people whose income is not withheld, or whose withholding is less than the estimated tax liability, submit a declaration for their estimated earnings for the year and make a payment each quarter.

A similar method is used by Japan, where income tax is collected by self-assessment unless it is withheld at the source. The income tax on wages, salaries, interest, and dividends is withheld at the source. Other kinds of incomes are subjected to the self-assessment system by which the taxpayers are required to make advance payments on July 31 and November 30 on the estimated payment. By March 15 of the following year they must complete the payment (final return). In view of the growth of the economy, the estimated incomes, and thus the tax liabilities, are systematically under-estimated, causing a lag between earning of incomes, other than wages, salaries, interest, and dividends and payments of the income tax on them.

DE FACTO TREATMENT OF INCOMES OF DIFFERENT ORIGIN

In analyzing how different types of incomes were taxed in each country, we must realize that the incomes reported by the tax authorities are normally quite different from those obtained from national accounts data. Therefore, it is important to examine the relationship between the incomes reported for taxation and those obtained from national accounts data. In this way estimates of the degree of erosion will be obtained for each type of income in each country and for the same countries over a period of time.

France

Table V-3 provides the distribution of income subjected to the progressive income tax for the period 1954-65. Wages and salaries accounted for a very large proportion—from 62.1 to 70.4 per cent—of the total taxed income; this proportion, which was reduced to 62.1 after the reform of 1959, has been increasing in recent years, reaching a level of 70 per cent in 1965. Among the other incomes, that from business is the most important averaging around 20 per cent. The trend for the share from this income has been downward during the last six years as shown in the table.

Table V-4 indicates the degree of erosion to which four major categories of income were subjected. In 1965, the last year for which this information is

TABLE V-3. PERCENTAGE DISTRIBUTION OF MAJOR CATEGORIES OF INCOME
SUBJECT TO THE INDIVIDUAL INCOME TAX, 1954-65

Categories of income	1954	1955	1956	1957	1958	1959	1960	1961	1962	1963	1964	1965
Wages and salaries	64.1	62.7	64.6	67.6	66.5	70.4	62.1	62.6	63.6	65.9	69.7	70.0
Business	23.5	23.9	22.5	19.9	21.4	18.3	24.8	23.2	22.4	20.6	19.5	18.4
Noncommercial activity	3.9	5.1	5.0	4.8	4.8	4.6	5.0	5.0	5.0	4.4	4.3	4.5
Movable capital	4.0	4.2	4.1	3.8	3.6	3.3	3.4	3.9	3.7	3.5	3.3	3.1
Real property	0.9	0.9	0.8	1.3	1.4	1.5	1.9	2.3	2.3	2.4	2.4	2.0
Others	3.6	3.2	3.0	2.6	2.3	1.9	2.8	3.0	3.0	3.2	0.8	2.0
Total	100.0	100.0	100.0	100.0	100.0	100.0	100.0	100.0	100.0	100.0	100.0	100.0

Sources: France, Ministère de l'Economie et des Finances, *Statistiques et Etudes Financières,* Supplement (Paris: Imprimerie Nationale, monthly); and Ministère de l'Economie et des Finances, *Renseignements Statistiques Relatifs aux Impôts Directs* (Paris: Imprimerie Nationale, 76e année).

TABLE V-4. MAJOR CATEGORIES OF INCOME FROM NATIONAL ACCOUNTS
AND FROM TAX DATA FOR FRANCE, 1955-65

(francs in billions)

Incomes	1955	1956	1957	1958	1959	1960	1961	1962	1963	1964	1965
Wages and salaries											
A. National accounts data[a]	55.28	62.49	70.43	81.79	89.53	98.81	109.25	122.31	140.18	155.76	168.15
B. Tax data	15.62	19.69	24.81	28.07	36.12	32.80	37.57	44.97	54.27	69.33	78.30
C. B as a % of A	28.26%	31.51%	35.23%	34.32%	40.34%	33.20%	34.39%	36.77%	38.71%	44.51%	46.57%
Income from real property											
A. National accounts data[a]	2.82	2.76	2.78	3.35	3.64	4.58	5.45	6.47	7.20	7.47	8.85
B. Tax data	0.22	0.25	0.46	0.59	0.75	1.00	1.40	1.66	2.01	2.39	2.27
C. B as a % of A	7.80%	9.06%	16.55%	17.61%	20.60%	21.83%	25.69%	25.66%	27.92%	32.00%	25.65%
Income from movable capital											
A. National accounts data[a]	6.00	6.54	7.37	7.97	8.36	8.89	9.38	10.33	10.71	11.15	13.07
B. Tax data	1.04	1.24	1.41	1.50	1.67	1.77	2.34	2.63	2.89	3.24	3.51
C. B as a % of A	17.33%	18.96%	19.13%	18.82%	19.98%	19.91%	24.95%	25.46%	26.98%	29.06%	26.85%
Income from business											
A. National accounts data[a]	39.39	42.94	47.87	56.31	58.36	66.60	67.27	76.00	79.59	83.20	86.77
B. Tax data	5.95	6.87	7.32	9.03	9.39	13.10	13.94	15.86	17.00	19.35	20.67
C. B as a % of A	15.11%	16.00%	15.29%	16.04%	16.09%	19.67%	20.72%	20.87%	21.36%	23.26%	23.82%

[a]Net of employers' contributions to social security.

Sources: See sources for Tables V-2 and V-3.

available, 46.57 per cent of wages and salaries as shown by the national accounts statistics were subjected to the progressive income tax. For the other types of incomes the percentages were: 25.65 for incomes from real property, 26.85 for incomes from movable property, and 23.82 for business income. Thus, each of these four types of income was subject to a substantial degree of erosion, but this erosion was much less serious for wages and salaries than for other incomes. To the extent that the erosion was mostly due to illegal evasion, this confirms the widespread credence that evasion of income taxes is more difficult for wage and salary earners. It also indicates that business incomes are the most difficult to control.

Table V-4 shows also the substantial progress which has been made in limiting the degree of erosion in each of these income categories: the percentage for wages and salaries increased from 28.26 in 1955 to 46.57 in 1965; that for income from real property increased from 7.8 to 32 in 1964 but decreased again to 25.65 in 1965; that for income from movable capital, from 17.33 to 29.06 in 1964 and 26.85 in 1965. The increase in the percentage for income from business was the lowest of all going from 15.11 to 23.82. This is important if it is true that business incomes are the ones most likely to be saved and reinvested because it would imply that the difference in the degree of erosion may have contributed to personal saving. In the absence of specific evidence this must remain a possibility.

If the personal income tax were strictly a proportional one, then the above information would tell us about the relative contribution of each type of income to the total income tax revenue. However, this tax is progressive, and the income distribution by size is not independent of the income allocation by type. Therefore, the average tax rate can be expected to differ from one type of income to another. Thus, it is only through a careful analysis of the allocation of each income bracket through the types of income that an estimate of the average tax rate by type of income can be obtained.

These estimates, together with the relative contribution of each type of income to the total tax payment are shown in Table V-5. The table shows large differences among the average tax rates on the different categories of reported income, and it indicates that the tax treatment of wages and salaries is much lighter than that of other kinds of incomes; the rate on incomes from financial investments (movable capital) appears particularly high. However, one must reckon with the problem of erosion since, as seen in Table V-4, the degree to which different incomes are eroded with respect to income taxation is very different. In order to get a more accurate picture of the real weight of the average rates on these incomes, one ought to relate the tax not to the reported income but to the estimates of those incomes obtained from national accounts statistics. When this is done (see the last column of Table V-5), the average rates which are obtained are much lower than those

THE INDIVIDUAL INCOME TAX

TABLE V-5. AVERAGE TAX RATE BY CATEGORY OF INCOME
FOR FRANCE, 1963

(percentages)

Sources of income	Total income reported by taxpayers	Contribution to individual income tax	Average tax rate on income reported[a]	Distribution of income from national accounts data	Average tax rate on national accounts estimates of incomes
Wages and salaries	65.9	48.3	11.0	56.8	4.2
Business[b]	22.0	29.8	18.7	{ 35.5	{
Noncommercial activities	4.4	9.0	24.6	n.a.	{ 5.4
Real property	2.5	3.1	n.a.	3.1	4.5
Movable capital	3.5	.6	29.0	4.8	7.9
Miscellaneous	1.7	2.2	12.0	n.a.	n.a.
Total	100.0	100.0	15.6	100.0	4.9

[a]These rates are not directly available from the French Tax Authorities. I have, however, developed a method that produces fairly accurate estimates. This method is described in detail in my dissertation, "The Structure of the Individual Income Tax in Major Industrial Countries" (Harvard, 1966).

[b]Includes agricultural income.

Sources: France, Ministère des Finances, *Statistiques et Etudes Financières*, Supplement (Paris: Imprimerie Nationale, monthly); O.E.C.D., *National Accounts Statistics, 1955-1964* (Paris: O.E.C.D., 1966).

reported in the third column of the table, and the differences among the rates
on different incomes which were quite substantial in the third column,
become much less important.

Germany

An analysis along the line followed for France is not possible for Germany
for lack of the necessary data, but we can attempt to estimate the imposition
of wages and salaries as compared with other types of incomes.

The statistical information is presented in Tables V-6 and V-7. Table V-6
gives the average income tax rate on wages and salaries for the period
1953-65; Table V-7 gives the same information for incomes from property
and enterprise going to household.

TABLE V-6. AVERAGE TAX RATES ON INCOMES FROM WAGES AND
SALARIES FOR GERMANY, 1953-65

(DM in billions)

Years	Wage tax	Income from wages and salaries		Average tax rate on wages and salaries	
		(a)	(b)	(a)	(b)
1953	3.74	65.77	59.40	5.68%	6.30%
1954	3.87	71.87	65.00	5.39	5.95
1955	4.40	81.95	73.94	5.37	5.95
1956	5.40	91.82	82.87	5.88	6.51
1957	5.29	100.52	89.70	5.26	5.90
1958	5.93	108.99	96.75	5.44	6.13
1959	5.86	116.83	103.88	5.01	5.64
1960	8.10	139.77	124.24	5.79	6.52
1961	10.45	157.18	140.11	6.64	7.45
1962	12.31	173.86	155.16	7.08	7.92
1963	13.84	186.53	166.50	7.41	8.31
1964	16.09	204.42	183.40	7.87	8.78
1965	16.74	224.70	202.70	7.54	8.26

Notes: (a) Includes employers' contributions to social insurance funds.
(b) Does not include employers' contributions to social insurance funds.

Sources: Germany, Deutsche Bundesbank, *Monthly Report* (Frankfurt); Statistical
Office of the European Communities, *General Statistical Bulletin* (Brussels: E.E.C.,
monthly).

In connection with these two tables it must be remembered that "taxes are
adjudicated on wage or salary incomes of DM24,000 or more, or on such
incomes of any amounts if there is additional nonwage income exceeding
DM600."[11] Therefore, while the income reported in Table V-6 is the whole
income from wages and salaries, the wage tax is not the whole tax on that

[11]Frederick G. Reuss, *Fiscal Policy for Growth without Inflation* (Baltimore: The
Johns Hopkins Press, 1963), p. 74.

TABLE V-7. AVERAGE TAX RATES ON INCOMES FROM PROPERTY AND
ENTERPRISE GOING TO HOUSEHOLDS FOR GERMANY, 1953-65

(DM in billions)

Years	Income from property and enterprise going to household	Assessed income tax	Capital yield tax	Total tax	Average tax rates on income from property and enterprise
1953	37.16	4.87	0.15	5.02	13.50%
1954	39.70	4.59	0.26	4.85	12.21
1955	45.89	4.35	0.34	4.69	10.22
1956	50.08	4.73	0.42	5.15	10.28
1957	53.66	5.88	0.48	6.36	11.85
1958	56.61	5.47	0.51	5.98	10.56
1959	61.38	7.32	0.83	8.15	13.27
1960	70.91	8.96	0.85	9.81	13.83
1961	74.68	10.82	0.98	11.80	15.80
1962	78.35	12.22	1.13	13.35	17.03
1963	81.71	13.45	1.14	14.59	17.94
1964	89.31	14.10	1.25	15.35	17.18
1965	94.80	14.80	1.35	16.15	17.04

Sources: Same as Table V-6.

income. Consequently, the average tax rates are affected downward. The opposite bias affects Table V-7 so that the average tax rates shown there are underestimated. These biases cannot be measured, but a comparison of the data in Table IV-3 with those in Table V-6 shows clearly that they cannot be very important. This comparison shows that in 1961 the wages and salaries subjected to the wage tax (DM129 billion) were more than 92 per cent of the wages and salaries reported by the national income accounts (DM140 billion). It is unlikely that more than a small fraction of the unaccounted 8 per cent was subjected to the adjudicated tax.

Two aspects of Tables V-6 and V-7 are of interest. One is the very substantial difference between the average tax rates on wages and salaries and those on other incomes. This difference ranged from a low of 3.77 percentage points in 1956 to a high of 9.63 in 1963. Since the incomes used are taken from the national accounts data, it is easy to realize how heavy these rates have become on incomes from property and enterprise.

Secondly, looking at the rates over the period under consideration one can divide that period in two parts: 1953-58, 1958-65. The first, which corresponds to what has been called the "period of normalization,"[12] is characterized by generally decreasing average tax rates, especially on incomes from property and enterprise going to households. The second period, or "period of overemployment"[13] is characterized by generally increasing average tax

[12]See Karl Häuser, "West Germany," N.B.E.R. and The Brookings Institution, *Foreign Tax Policies and Economic Growth* (New York: Columbia University Press, 1966), p. 109.

[13]*Ibid.*, p. 111.

rates: From 1958 to 1965 the rate for wages and salaries increased from 6.13 to 8.26. It was, however, for the other incomes that the increase was particularly large—over 7 percentage points in seven years! Furthermore, over the same period, there was a substantial increase in the share of wages and salaries in the national income—from 60.5 per cent in 1958 to 66 per cent in 1965 (see Table V-2). Therefore, using Dosser's terminology, the German income tax has become, since 1958, definitively dynamic-regressive.[14]

If it is true that the marginal propensity to save is higher for incomes other than wages and salaries, these two developments should have had a noticeable effect on the share of household saving in the disposable income. Between 1958 and 1963, there was a decrease in the percentage of disposable income saved from 14.2 to 12.3. A correlation of personal saving and personal income taxes, both expressed as percentages of household incomes—i.e., $\frac{Sp}{Yp} = a + b\frac{Tp}{Yp}$—for the period 1955-63 proved to be negative and significant at the 1 per cent level ($r = -.85$).

Perhaps the elimination of wages and salaries and the wage tax from the elements of the above correlation would make the impact of income taxes on saving even more obvious. Let us ignore saving out of wages and salaries and assume that all household saving comes from other incomes. Then, the income taxes which ought to be relevant are those on incomes from property and enterprise. Table V-8 shows the average income tax rates and the average

TABLE V-8. TAXES ON INCOMES FROM PROPERTY AND ENTERPRISE AND TOTAL PERSONAL SAVINGS AS PERCENTAGES, 1958-63

Years	Taxes as % of income	Saving as % of income
1958	10.56	40.98
1959	13.27	39.75
1960	13.83	39.98
1961	15.80	38.22
1962	17.03	36.12
1963	17.94	37.34

Source: Same as Table V-6.

saving rates so calculated. There is no doubt that there is a high, negative relationship as shown in Figure V-1. Of course, one must always be aware of the possibility that the decline in saving may have been due to some factor other than the tax increase. However, that increase was so large that it would be strange if it were not the basic factor.

[14]D. Dosser, "Tax Incidence and Growth," *The Economic Journal,* Vol. LXXI, September 1961.

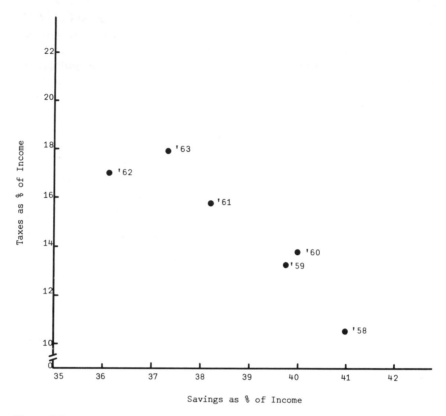

Figure V-I. Relationship Between Taxes on Incomes From Property, Enterprise, and Personal Saving, Germany, 1958-63

Italy

The analysis of the treatment of incomes from different origins is simplified, to a certain extent, by the schedular character of the Italian major income tax. It should be recalled that in Italy incomes are taxed by the *Imposta di Ricchezza Mobile,* which is the most important, and also by the *Imposta Complementare Progressiva,* the tax on the total income of the taxpayer.

It will be remembered from Chapter II that the *Imposta di Ricchezza Mobile* is a schedular tax with four major schedules for four different types of income. The four schedules are, briefly: A for incomes from capital; B for incomes from commercial, industrial, and speculative operations. This schedule applies also to the income of the corporations thus removing from the *Imposta di Ricchezza Mobile* its strictly personal character, and making the burden of this tax on individuals appear heavier than it is. Schedule C_1 concerns the income from independent professions and other "autonomous" work and also the income from small, family-type establishments. Schedule C_2, finally, deals with incomes from wages and salaries, pensions, allowances, and transfers. Under the jurisdiction of the *Ricchezza Mobile* falls also a tax on income from land which is no longer of any significance.

Table V-9 gives the percentage distribution of the revenues from *Ricchezza Mobile* according to the four schedules and the land tax. For this tax, taxable income which in 1954-55 amounted to 2,173 billion lire, by 1962 had increased by 174.5 per cent reaching a level of 5,065 billion lire. The tax imposed on this income increased from 223 billion lire in 1954-55 to 580.7 billion lire in 1962. This implies a decrease of the average tax rate from 10.2 to 9.7.

Schedule B, which is largely the income of incorporated businesses, accounted in 1963 for 50.5 per cent of the total revenues from the *Ricchezza Mobile*. Schedule A accounted for 13.5 per cent and schedules C_1 and C_2 accounted for 4.6 per cent and 30.9 per cent respectively. The corresponding percentages for 1954-55 were: 65.7 for B, 4.4 for A, 3.9 for C_1, and 25.0 for C_2. There was, therefore, a decrease in the relative contribution of schedule B and increases in the contributions of the other three schedules.

The national accounts of Italy do not provide the breakdown necessary to evaluate the share of national income which goes to each of these four categories. The share of wages and salaries in the national income was 50.8 per cent in 1955 and 58.7 per cent in 1963. Since the tax payments out of wages and salaries (schedule C_2) were respectively 25 per cent and 28.1 per cent, it cannot be said a priori that the personal income tax was discriminat-

TABLE V-9. DISTRIBUTION OF REVENUES FROM *RICCHEZZA MOBILE*
BY SCHEDULE, 1954-55 to 1963

(percentages)

	A	B	C_1	C_2	Land tax	Total[a]
1954-55	4.4	65.7	3.9	25.0	1.0	100.0
1955-56	7.0	63.6	3.7	24.8	0.9	100.0
1956-57	8.2	61.5	3.8	25.7	0.8	100.0
1957-58	8.6	59.7	3.9	27.1	0.7	100.0
1958-59	9.4	58.1	4.0	27.9	0.6	100.0
1960	11.2	55.9	4.2	28.2	0.5	100.0
1961	11.2	55.9	4.5	28.0	0.4	100.0
1962	12.1	55.1	4.5	28.1	0.3	100.0
1963	13.5	50.5	4.6	30.9	0.4	100.0

[a]May not add up to 100 because of rounding.

Source: Italy, Ministero delle Finanze, *L'Attività Tributaria dal 1954 al 1964* (Rome: Istituto Poligrafico dello Stato, 1964), Vol. II.

ing against those incomes. On the other hand, one must be cautious not to conclude that there was discrimination in favor of wages and salaries since these were normally quite low. The inclusion of schedule B is misleading in view of the fact that this is mostly corporate income. If this income is not considered and one looks back at Table V-9, then the comparison of the revenues from C_2 (25 per cent of the total in 1954-55, and 30.9 per cent in 1963) with those from A and C (8.3 per cent in 1954-55 and 18.1 per cent in 1963) gives a clear indication that, although all incomes are taxed with very low rates in Italy, the effective rates on incomes other than those from wages and salaries are extremely low. Since the nominal rates on these incomes are much higher than on wages and salaries, and since the size of the exemptions are somewhat lower, the only explanation has to be found in the degree of "erosion" (in this case "evasion" is a more appropriate word) of the different types of income.

In fact the ratio of the (taxed) base to the national income was 21.9 per cent in 1954 and 30.7 per cent in 1962. At the same time, the share of taxed wages and salaries was 22 per cent in 1954 and 33 per cent in 1962. This is quite remarkable if one remembers that this was income actually taxed. In other words, in spite of the fact that incomes other than wages and salaries are normally received by people whose average incomes can be expected to exceed substantially those of people who work for wages and salaries, a smaller share of the former is subjected to taxation under the *Ricchezza Mobile* schedule.

Table V-10 gives the total picture of the effective taxation of reported income for the four schedules of the *Ricchezza Mobile*. It shows that the average tax rate has been increasing for the incomes of schedule A and B and decreasing for those of C_1; for C_2 there had not been any significant change up to 1962.

A comparison of the effective rates on reported incomes shows great differences among the various schedules with A and B being levied with the highest rates and C_1 and C_2 with the lowest. These rates reflect the differences in the nominal rates, but, as argued above, the different degree of evasion renders these differences much less significant than they appear.

The relatively small contribution of professional and artisan incomes (C_1) should also be noticed. Schedule C_1, it must be remembered, includes not only people in nonsalaried professions but also small business owners, shopkeepers, small traders, and similar occupations. All the evidence which is available suggests that those with incomes of the C_1 category find it easiest to evade the tax. Above all, this group, because of its political power, has always succeeded in getting a very favorable legal tax treatment which is obvious from Table V-10. Their total contribution to these revenues has been around 4 per cent which is surely much less than their share of the personal income.

TABLE V-10. TAXABLE INCOME, TAX, AND TAX PAYMENTS AS PERCENTAGES OF TAXABLE INCOME FOR
THE *RICCHEZZA MOBILE*, 1954-55 to 1963

(lire in billions)

Years	A			B			C_1			C_2		
	Taxable income	Tax	Average tax rate	Taxable income	Tax	Average tax rate	Taxable income	Tax	Average tax rate	Taxable income	Tax	Average tax rate
1954-55	44.3	9.7	21.9%	834.2	146.0	17.5%	116.3	8.7	7.4%	1,154.1	55.6	4.8%
1955-56	81.9	18.0	21.9	913.1	163.2	17.8	132.7	9.5	7.2	1,470.8	63.8	4.4
1956-57	110.2	24.2	21.9	1,042.0	181.3	17.3	180.2	11.2	6.2	1,775.2	75.8	4.2
1957-58	126.0	28.4	22.5	1,134.6	197.5	17.4	195.1	13.1	6.7	2,014.3	89.7	4.4
1958-59	157.9	34.7	21.9	1,240.8	214.1	17.2	223.8	14.8	6.6	2,351.9	103.0	4.3
1960	212.4	48.2	22.6	1,342.4	241.9	18.0	277.0	18.1	6.5	2,779.2	122.1	4.3
1961	243.3	55.2	23.5	1,513.5	275.9	18.2	348.1	22.2	6.3	3,062.0	138.4	4.5
1962	283.9	70.1	24.6	1,693.4	319.9	18.8	474.7	25.9	5.4	3,493.1	163.0	4.6
1963	n.a.	89.3	n.a.	n.a.	334.2	n.a.	n.a.	30.8	n.a.	n.a.	204.5	n.a.

Source: Arranged from data in Italy, Ministero delle Finanze, *L'Attivita' Tributaria dal 1954 al 1964* (Rome: Istituto Poligrafico dello Stato, 1964), Vol. I.

There are some glaring indications of the fiscal ethics of this group. In 1962, 174,500 taxpayers voluntarily submitted a declaration and reported an income of 144.4 billion lire. The tax authority, however, was able to "discover" almost ten times that many and to increase the taxable income from 144.4 to 474.7 billion lire.[15] The privileged treatment of this group, together with the facility of evasion has at least two bad consequences: first, it encourages very high standards of living among many of this group with consequent "demonstration effects" which are particularly important, since the members of this group are pace setters in consumption; second, it encourages a form of activity which is really an anachronism in a developed country. The number of small shops in Italy exceeds by far that justified by an efficient system.[16] This tremendous proliferation of small traders has led to abnormally high costs of distribution, absorbing some of the productivity gains which have been quite remarkable in the Italian manufacturing and agricultural sectors.

This situation is bound to lead to trouble. As long as the large pool of unemployed workers was available, the pressure on wages was not too great. This permitted the Italian economy to develop at a very fast rate with very small increases in wholesale prices and wages. However, by 1961 some bottlenecks developed in the labor market, and prompted by what has been called a "consumption euphoria," demands on wages became more insistent. Of the increase in national income between 1961 and 1962, 75.7 per cent went to wages and salaries; of that between 1962 and 1963, 96.5 per cent went to wages and salaries; of that between 1963 and 1964 the share going to wages and salaries was 72.5. In these three years—which were prosperity years—the share of national income going to wages and salaries increased more than for the whole decade of the 1950's, going from 52.3 per cent 1961 to 59.9 per cent in 1964.[17]

It is possible to argue that given the social and political conditions which exist now in Italy, there is bound to be a redistribution of income among the various income classes. If such a redistribution is not brought about by a progressive tax system, it will be brought about by other means (increasing

[15]It should be mentioned that a law of January 11, 1951 obliges all income earners to report their income annually. Lists of taxpayers, called "roles," are prepared every year by the Tax Authority and made available to the offices in charge of tax collection.

[16]See Richard H. Holton, "Economic Development and the Growth of Trade Sector in Italy," *Banca Nazionale del Lavoro Quarterly Review,* September 1962, pp. 240-57. Holton talks about a "retailing population explosion."

[17]For an analysis of the role that the tax system of Italy has played in the growth process of the last decade, see Vito Tanzi, "La Struttura del Sistema Fiscale Italiano: Un Confronto Internazionale," *Rivista Internazionale di Scienze Economiche e Commerciali,* Anno VIII, No. 6, 1966.

takeover on the part of an already large public sector, increasing labor pressure, etc.).[18]

This section has centered on the *Ricchezza Mobile,* because this is by far the most important income tax in Italy and because there is no way of allocating the revenues from the other income tax—the *Imposta Complementare*—among different kinds of incomes. However, the revenues from this tax are so low that its omission from the discussion is hardly serious.

Table V-11 shows the main findings of this section.

TABLE V-11. INCOME TAX TREATMENT OF WAGES AND SALARIES
AND OTHER INCOMES IN ITALY, 1962

		(percentages)
	Wages and salaries	Other incomes
Per cent of incomes reported in national income accounts actually taxed	33.0	27.7
Per cent of taxed income	58.8	41.2
Per cent of tax revenue	28.2	71.8
Average tax on taxed income	4.6	16.0
Average tax on national income	1.5	4.7

Sources: Tables V-9 and V-10 and text.

United Kingdom

In Table V-12, I have calculated for several selected fiscal years the ratio of the "net produce of tax"[19] on each schedule to the "actual income."[20] It is important to realize that the table concerns only the "income tax" and thus does not account for the surtax which is particularly heavy on investment income. In spite of this distortion, it gives a striking picture of the different incidence of the tax among incomes of different origin.

Schedule A and C which are taxed with rates of close to 40 per cent, represent respectively income from real property (buildings, lands, etc.) and "interest from British government and overseas government and public authority securities taxed by deduction." Schedule D concerns profits from business, professions, and certain interests. This is predominantly profits of

[18]See *ibid.* for a discussion of this point.

[19]Defined as "the estimated ultimate yield from the tax assessed in the year, whether actually collected in that year or later, after deducting all discharges and remissions and setting off all repayments."

[20]This is defined as "the statutory income of persons above the effective exemption limit computed in accordance with the provisions of the Income Tax Acts." The tax is actually imposed on the taxable income which is "the actual income less earned income relief and other personal allowances and deductions."

corporations; however, in 1962-63, 21.5 per cent was income of individuals and 10.5 per cent was income of partnerships.[21] The average tax rate on individuals was 14.5 per cent; on partnerships it was 17.9 per cent.[22]

TABLE V-12. NET PRODUCE OF TAX AS A PERCENTAGE OF "ACTUAL INCOME," SELECTED FISCAL YEARS, THE UNITED KINGDOM

(percentages)

Income categories	Average tax			
	1958-59	1959-60	1962-63	1963-64
A	36.4	32.8	32.4	38.6
C	39.3	35.9	36.2	36.6
D	27.7	22.9	23.3	22.5
E	8.2	8.0	9.3	8.9

Source: Great Britain, Board of Inland Revenue, *Report of the Commissioners of Her Majesty's Inland Revenue* (London: H.M.S.O., several years).

Finally, schedule E, which represents income from employment, is taxed with average rates which are very low when compared with those on the other incomes. These rates confirm once again that the British income tax is far too heavy on incomes from sources other than wages and salaries and relatively low on the latter incomes.

As noted above, the estimates in Table V-12 concern only the income tax. When the surtax is considered, the differential burden of taxation between incomes from wages and salaries and incomes from other sources becomes even more accentuated. It is necessary to recall that, because of the various exemptions provided to "earned" incomes, most of the burden of the surtax falls on incomes other than wages and salaries. Only 25 per cent of the national income is made up of incomes other than wages and salaries, which further emphasizes the disproportionate tax burden on that sector.

Unfortunately the breakdown of the data on the surtax does not make it possible to allocate the revenues according to the four schedules of Table V-12. The following conclusions can be drawn: In the last few years, the revenues from the surtax were less than .5 per cent of the incomes from wages and salaries, while they were over 6 per cent of the other incomes.[23] Furthermore, the breakdown of the income subjected to the surtax between "earned" and "investment" suggests clearly that the share of "earned" to

[21] See Great Britain, Board of Inland Revenue, *Report of the Commissioners of Her Majesty's Inland Revenue, 1964* (London: H.M.S.O., 1965), p. 53.

[22] *Ibid.*

[23] Estimated from Tables 22 and 46 of Great Britain, Central Statistical Office, *National Income and Expenditure, 1964* (London: H.M.S.O., 1965).

total has been decreasing which implies that the surtax has been becoming heavier on investment incomes.[24]

Table V-13 combines the income tax with the surtax for wages and salaries and other incomes. The incomes shown in the table come from national accounts data and thus are different from the taxable incomes. The difference in the average tax rate between incomes from wages and salaries and other incomes is quite considerable. With respect to the taxes on incomes from wages and salaries, by far the largest part of them come from middle and higher salaries since most of the lower salaries seldom pay any income taxes.

The table also indicates that the average tax rate on wages and salaries has been increasing from around 6 per cent in 1955 to 9.58 per cent in 1965. On the other hand, the average rate on the other incomes has remained substantially unchanged. The two trends combined have resulted in a generally increasing ratio of the total taxes on income to total personal income.

TABLE V-13. TAXATION OF INCOMES FROM WAGES AND SALARIES
AND OF OTHER PERSONAL INCOMES FOR THE
UNITED KINGDOM, 1955-65

(£ in millions)

Years	Income from wages and salaries	Income tax and surtax	Average tax rate	Income from other sources	Income tax and surtax	Average tax rate
1955	11,244	681	6.06%	2,872	649	22.6%
1956	12,257	783	6.39	2,956	669	22.6
1957	12,958	895	6.91	3,111	707	22.7
1958	13,460	977	7.26	3,348	719	21.5
1959	14,987	1,007	7.15	3,678	769	20.9
1960	15,144	1,147	7.57	3,985	854	21.4
1961	16,372	1,312	8.01	4,295	947	22.0
1962	17,254	1,464	8.48	4,452	1,005	22.6
1963	18,120	1,447	7.99	4,733	1,060	22.4
1964	19,536	1,636	8.37	4,948	1,114	22.5
1965	20,965	2,008	9.58	n.a.	1,242	n.a.

Sources: Great Britain, Central Statistical Office, *National Income and Expenditure, 1966* (London: H.M.S.O.), Table 51, Table 2; and O.E.C.D., *National Accounts Statistics, 1955-1964* (Paris: O.E.C.D., 1966).

Japan

Table V-14, dealing with wages and salaries, shows the average tax rate with respect to the total compensation of employees (C/A), the average tax rate with respect to the taxed income (C/B), and the extent to which the compensation of the employees is subjected to taxation (B/A). The erosion of

[24]In 1960-61, earned income was £1,265 million while investment income was £760 million. In 1962-63, earned income was £845 million while investment income was £805 million. See *Inland Revenue Report, op. cit.,* p. 99.

THE INDIVIDUAL INCOME TAX

TABLE V-14. INCOME TAX ON WAGES AND SALARIES IN JAPAN,
1954-65

(yen in billions)

Years	Wages and salaries (A)	Taxed income (B)	Tax (C)	C/A	C/B	B/A
1954	2,983	2,196	197	6.6%	8.9%	73.6%
1955	3,180	2,286	189	5.9	8.3	71.9
1956	3,612	2,545	205	5.7	8.0	70.5
1957	4,075	2,892	160	3.9	5.5	71.0
1958	4,383	3,193	155	3.5	4.9	72.8
1959	4,935	3,481	166	3.4	4.8	70.5
1960	5,776	4,311	221	3.8	5.1	74.6
1961	6,925	5,384	266	3.8	4.9	77.7
1962	8,162	6,693	312	3.8	4.7	82.0
1963	9,502	7,944	391	4.1	4.9	83.6
1964	10,994	9,404	495	4.5	5.3	85.5
1965	12,445	10,559	560	4.5	5.3	84.8

Source: Japan, Ministry of Finance, Tax Bureau, *Major Statistics of Taxation in Japan* ([available only in Japanese] Tokyo: 1966).

this tax base for income tax purposes was very limited. For the period covered by the data, the ratio of taxed income to the income received from dependent work was never lower than 70 per cent. Since 1962, it has been well above 80 per cent. The average tax rate on the total income received from wages and salaries was around 4 per cent.

Table V-15 provides the same type of information as the first table for business income. The latter is divided in two categories: agricultural income and nonagricultural business income. The table shows that only a small share of this income is taxed. This is particularly true for agricultural income for which the percentage taxed has been falling and was as low as 6 per cent in 1965. Because of this, and also because the average tax rate on taxed income was very low—normally between 2 and 3 per cent—the average tax rate on agricultural income was extremely low; in 1965 it was only 1 per cent.

For nonagricultural business income, the share which was taxed was close to 30 per cent and the average tax on the total income was over 2 per cent; thus, the average rate on the taxed income was more than 8 per cent, which was somewhat higher than the average rate on income from wages and salaries.

Information on taxation of incomes other than wages and salaries and business incomes is not available in the official data. Property incomes are included in the "other incomes" category. In Table V-16 I have estimated the average tax rate on these incomes by subtracting incomes from wages and salaries and business from total reported personal incomes. By subtracting the tax on the latter from that of the former we arrive at the tax on other incomes. The average tax rate on other incomes can then be calculated by

TABLE V-15. INCOME TAX ON INDIVIDUAL BUSINESS INCOME IN JAPAN, 1954-65

(yen in billions)

Years	Agricultural income						Other business					
	Total income (A)	Taxed income (B)	Tax (C)	C/A	C/B	B/A	Total income (A)	Taxed income (B)	Tax (C)	C/A	C/B	B/A
1954	964	178	84	9%	47%	18.5%	1,228	390	44	3.6%	11.4%	34.4%
1955	1,130	245	111	10	45	21.7	1,302	369	37	2.8	10.0	28.4
1956	1,056	172	69	7	40	16.3	1,470	415	45	3.1	10.0	28.2
1957	1,076	191	59	6	31	17.7	1,537	442	37	2.4	8.4	28.7
1958	1,091	177	49	5	28	16.2	1,452	427	30	2.0	7.0	29.4
1959	1,162	142	33	3	23	12.2	1,582	462	32	2.0	7.0	29.2
1960	1,215	145	36	3	25	12.0	1,811	551	44	2.4	7.9	30.4
1961	1,307	75	22	2	29	5.7	2,171	587	47	2.2	8.0	27.0
1962	1,466	97	27	2	27	6.6	2,368	666	52	2.2	7.8	28.1
1963	1,575	103	29	2	29	6.5	2,681	769	62	2.3	8.0	28.7
1964	1,734	121	34	2	28	7.0	2,982	870	73	2.4	8.3	29.2
1965	1,857	112	21	1	19	6.0	3,255	929	79	2.4	8.5	28.5

Source: Japan, Ministry of Finance, Tax Bureau, *Major Statistics of Taxation in Japan ([available only in Japanese] Tokyo: 1966).*

TABLE V-16. AVERAGE TAX RATES ON INCOMES OTHER THAN WAGES
AND SALARIES AND BUSINESS INCOMES IN JAPAN, 1954-65

(yen in billions)

Years	(1) Total personal income	(2) Wages, salaries, and business incomes	(3) Other incomes	(4) Tax on (1)	(5) Tax on (2)	(6) (4-5)	Average tax rate on other incomes
1954	5,670	5,175	495	291	249	42	8.5%
1955	6,192	5,613	579	278	237	41	7.2
1956	6,784	6,137	647	303	257	46	7.7
1957	7,411	6,689	722	258	203	55	7.6
1958	7,751	6,926	825	249	190	59	7.1
1959	8,674	7,679	995	281	202	79	8.0
1960	9,990	8,802	1,188	392	268	124	10.4
1961	11,776	10,404	1,372	487	315	172	12.5
1962	13,553	11,995	1,558	574	367	207	13.3
1963	15,530	13,758	1,772	687	455	232	13.1
1964	17,689	15,709	1,980	845	571	274	13.8
1965	19,794	17,556	2,238	990	642	348	15.5

Source: Calculated from data from Japan, Ministry of Finance, Tax Bureau, *Major Statistics of Taxation in Japan* ([available only in Japanese] Tokyo: 1966).

dividing tax revenues by the other income totals. This rate has been rising from a low of 7.1 per cent in 1958 to 15.5 per cent in 1965.

SUMMARY AND CONCLUSIONS

In the first part of this chapter, we saw how and why some countries discriminate in favor of incomes from dependent work. One of the reasons given for the preferential treatment of wage and salary earners was their alleged inability to evade taxation; in those countries where evasion is easy, a nondiscriminatory legal treatment of these incomes may result in actual discrimination. The first objective of the chapter was to analyze why the evasion of taxes on wages and salaries is more difficult than the evasion of taxes on other incomes. The second part analyzed the empirical evidence on the above issues.

The results of a country by country analysis supported the common belief that it is more difficult to evade taxes on wages and salaries than on other incomes. In France, around 70 per cent of the income subjected to the progressive income tax was wages and salaries. In 1965 the ratio of the reported income to the national income by type of income was much higher for wages and salaries than for any other major income category. It was 46.6 per cent for wages and salaries, 25.7 per cent for incomes from real property, 26.9 per cent for incomes from movable capital, and 23.8 per cent for incomes from business.

In Italy, reported wages and salaries were 33 per cent of their counterpart in the national accounts while all the other incomes combined were 27.7 per cent. In Germany, wages and salaries reported for taxation in 1961 were 92 per cent of their equivalent in the national accounts. Unfortunately, the reported income was not available for the other income categories, but the amount of taxes levied on these incomes was quite substantial making it unlikely that the reported income could have been low relative to its possible maximum. The United Kingdom's situation appears to be quite similar to the German since most incomes, regardless of their origin, are reported for taxation.

In Japan, a very high percentage of wages and salaries is reported (around 84 per cent in recent years), but a relatively low percentage of the other incomes (6 per cent for agricultural incomes and 28.5 per cent for the other business incomes) is reported. In the United States, most incomes are reported for taxation but the percentage for wages and salaries is somewhat higher than for the other incomes (87 per cent against 60 per cent).

These differential degrees of erosion among the different incomes have a lot to do with determining the average tax rate on each type of income. The main interest does not center on the reported incomes but on those from the national accounts (Table V-17). For France, the average tax rate estimated in relation to the reported income was 15.6 per cent, while in relation to personal income, it was only 4.9 per cent. For the specific incomes, the rates in relation to reported incomes were quite high (11 per cent for wages and salaries, 18.7 per cent for business income, 24.6 per cent for professional income, 29 per cent for movable wealth, and 12 per cent for other miscellaneous incomes), but in relation to the estimates from the national accounts data, they were much lower.

In Germany, even though the tax revenues are related to national accounts estimates of income, it becomes clear how much heavier the German tax is than the French. The difference is not so large for wages and salaries as it is for the other incomes; for the latter, the effective average tax rate in Germany was at least three times as high as for France.

In Italy too one finds a remarkable divergence between tax rates related to reported incomes and those related to actual incomes. For the total income, the rate goes from 9.7 per cent to 3 per cent while the rate for wages and salaries declines from 4.6 per cent to 1.5 per cent, and that for other incomes from 16 per cent to 4.7 per cent.

In the United Kingdom the effective rates related to the national accounts data are 10 per cent for total income, 8 per cent for wages and salaries, and 22.4 per cent for the other incomes.

TABLE V-17. AVERAGE TAX RATES IN RELATION TO REPORTED INCOME
AND NATIONAL ACCOUNTS ESTIMATES, 1963

(percentages)

Countries	Wages and salaries	Business income	Professional income	Real property	Movable wealth	Miscellaneous	Total
France							
Reported Income	11.0	18.7	24.6	n.a.	29.0	12.0	15.6
National Accounts	4.2	5.4	n.a.	4.5	7.9	n.a.	4.9
Germany							
Reported Income	7.1[a]	n.a.	n.a.	n.a.	n.a.	n.a.	n.a.
National Accounts	8.3	←			17.9		→	10.6
Italy							
Reported Income[b]	4.6	18.8	5.4	n.a.	24.6	n.a.	9.7
National Accounts	1.6	←			4.7		→	3.0
United Kingdom							
Reported Income	9.1	n.a.	n.a.	n.a.	n.a.	n.a.	n.a.
National Accounts	8.0	←			22.4		→	10.0
Japan							
Reported Income	4.9	7.5	←	13.1			→	8.1
National Accounts	4.5	1.5	n.a.	n.a.	n.a.	n.a.	n.a.

[a]1961.

[b]1962 for *Ricchezza Mobile*.

Source: See text and tables in Chapter V.

VI

EROSION OF THE INDIVIDUAL INCOME TAX BASE

For any one year, the relationship between the individual income tax revenue and the gross national product of a country can be written in the form of an identity as follows:

$$\frac{T}{GNP} = \frac{T}{TI} \times \frac{TI}{GNP}$$

where T stands for the revenues from the individual income tax and TI for taxable income (taxable in de facto rather than de jure sense[1]). Thus a change in T/GNP may be caused by either a change in T/TI or in the relationship between taxable income and GNP that is between the base of the income tax and the GNP.

I will call erosion the divergence between the gross national product and the income tax base (or TI). Literally, erosion implies a dynamic process;[2] however, the term is used here solely to describe that divergence that may, or may not, be increasing over time. This divergence is the result of several factors, some of which depend on the tax legislation of the countries with their inevitable deductions, exemptions, and their particular treatment of some specific incomes. Others depend on the institutional organization of the country, such as the importance of the corporate sector and the dividend policies of the corporations, the size of depreciation, the importance of the public sector, and other similar factors. Still others are connected with the tax morality of the taxpayers or, perhaps more importantly, with the opportunities for evasion.

Only for the United States and the United Kingdom would it have been possible to describe the step by step process of erosion; for the other

---

[1] If TI stood for taxable income in a de jure sense, the T/GNP would not be the actual but the potential burden given the nominal structure of the tax.

[2] That is the way in which Pechman has used the term for his analysis of this process in the United States. See J. A. Pechman, "Erosion of the Individual Income Tax," *National Tax Journal,* Vol. 10, No. 1, March 1957, pp. 1-25.

countries this information could not be found. Thus, for the sake of homogeneity, the intermediate steps are skipped and the analysis concentrates on
the final results.

EMPIRICAL EVIDENCE ON THE EROSION OF THE BASE

General Evidence

Table VI-1 provides the relationship between taxable income, personal
income, and the gross national product for four countries. Taxable income in
the table is the income actually taxed, and, thus, it is net of personal exemptions and other legal deductions. For this reason Japan and Germany could
not be included since the data available on taxable income for them are gross
of those exemptions and deductions.

TABLE VI-1. RELATIONSHIP BETWEEN TAXABLE INCOME, PERSONAL
INCOME, AND GNP FOR FOUR COUNTRIES, 1963

Countries	TI	Y_p	GNP	TI/Y_p	Y_p/GNP	TI/GNP
	national currencies, billions			percentages		
France	82.4	346.2	391.8	23.8	88.4	21.0
Italy[d]	5,965[a]	19,423[e]	24,789	30.7	78.4	24.1
	4,272[b]			21.9		17.2
	2,909[c]			15.0		11.7
United Kingdom[f]	10.4	24.1	28.7	43.2	84.0	36.2
United States	209.1	464.8	589.2	45.0	78.9	35.5

[a]Total taxable income for *Ricchezza Mobile*.

[b]Taxable income for Schedules A, C_1, and C_2 (i.e., without business incomes).

[c]Taxable income for *Imposta Complementare*.

[d]1962.

[e]National income.

[f]Taxable income 1962-63. Includes company income.

Sources: O.E.C.D., *National Accounts Statistics, 1955-1964* (Paris, 1966); for
France: Ministère de l'Economie et des Finances, *Statistiques et Etudes Financières,*
Supplement (Paris: Imprimerie Nationale); for Italy: Ministero delle Finanze, *L'Attività*
Tributaria dal 1954 al 1964 (Rome: Istituto Poligrafico dello Stato, 1964); for the
United Kingdom: Board of Inland Revenue, *Report of the Commissioners of Her*
Majesty's Inland Revenue (London: H.M.S.O., 1965); for the United States: Internal
Revenue Service, *Statistics of Income* (Washington, D. C., G.P.O., 1966).

There is considerable erosion in each of the countries. The United States in
1963 suffered least from erosion with a tax base equal to 35.5 per cent of the
gross national product and 45 per cent of the personal income. Next is the

United Kingdom with a base equal to 36.2 and 43.2 per cent respectively in relation to the gross national product and the personal income.[3]

The degree of erosion in Latin countries, is much larger. It must be recalled that France does not provide personal exemptions since very low incomes are not taxed (although once the income becomes taxable, it is taxed in its entirety). Therefore, in a way the percentages which are reported are overestimated. When compared with reported incomes (gross of the exemptions for the United States and the United Kingdom) the differences are much greater.

For Italy the table shows three different estimates: one for the *Ricchezza Mobile* without adjustment, one for the *Ricchezza Mobile* adjusted for the income of corporations, and one for the *Imposta Complementare*. The degree of erosion increases greatly between the first and the third of these estimates. This is what one would expect since large companies taxed with schedule B can evade the taxes to a much lesser degree than the others, and since, in general, it is harder to evade taxes on incomes subjected to the *Ricchezza Mobile* than on those subjected to the *Imposta Complementare*. Furthermore, when incomes are subjected to the latter tax, the exemptions provided are much higher; the consequence of the combination of high exemptions and high evasion is that only 11.7 per cent of the gross national product of Italy is subjected to the progressive, global income tax.

Since the corporate sector is more important in the United States and in the United Kingdom,[4] and since not all profits earned in this sector are distributed, one would expect the personal income tax base to differ most from the gross national product in these two countries than in Italy and France.

Enough data is available for Germany and Japan to justify an estimation of their erosion. In Table VI-2, the relationship between the reported income, personal income, and the gross national product is shown for five countries. Here the data for France are the same as in the first table; but for the United Kingdom and the United States, reported income has replaced taxed income. For Germany, the data refer to wages and salaries only.

Considering the ratio of the reported income to the personal income, there appears to be very little difference between the United States, the United Kingdom, and Japan. For Germany, comparative data are not available.

---

[3]The estimates for the United Kingdom are biased upward since the income of companies is included.

[4]The *Report of the Committee on Turnover Taxation* estimates that "in 1960 some 70 per cent of trading profits in the private sector of the economy in the United Kingdom were earned by companies, and some 30 per cent by individuals and partnerships . . . only some 30-40 per cent of trading profits are earned by companies in Germany and France." See Great Britain, *Report of the Committee on Turnover Taxation* (London: H.M.S.O., 1964), p. 10.

TABLE VI-2. RELATIONSHIP BETWEEN REPORTED INCOME,
PERSONAL INCOME (Y_p), AND GNP FOR FIVE COUNTRIES, 1963

Countries	RI	Y_p	GNP	RI/Y_p	Y_p/GNP	RI/GNP
	national currencies, billions			percentages		
France	82.4	346.2	391.8	23.8	88.4	21.0
Germany	129.0[a]	139.8[a]	326.2	92.3	n.a.	n.a.
Japan	11,989	15,964	22,454	75.1	71.1	53.4
United Kingdom	18.1[b]	24.1	28.7	75.1	84.0	63.1
United States	368.8[c]	464.8	589.2	79.3	78.9	62.6

[a] Wages and salaries only, for 1961.

[b] "Actual Income" for the fiscal year 1962-63. Does not include company income.

[c] Adjusted Gross Income.

Sources: See sources to Table VI-1 and, for Germany: Federal Office of Statistics, *Statistical Yearbook, 1966* (West Baden: 1966); for Japan: Ministry of Finance, Tax Bureau, *Major Statistics of Taxation in Japan* ([available only in Japanese] Tokyo: 1965).

However, in view of the very high share of reported wages and salaries and of the very high income taxes collected from other incomes in spite of relatively low rates, it is safe to conclude that the erosion could not be much higher here than in the other three countries and, conceivably, it might be even lower.

When these four countries are compared with France, their ratios appear to be strikingly high, further proof of the substantial evasion that occurs in that country. A comparison with Italy gives similar results.

The ratio of the personal income to the gross national product varies from country to country; thus, when reported (or taxed) income is taken as a percentage of the latter rather than the former, that percentage decreases significantly in some countries. In Japan for example, Y_p/GNP is only 71.1 per cent as compared with 84 per cent in the United Kingdom. Therefore, while these two countries have the same RI/Y_p (75.1), their RI/GNP is somewhat different: 63.1 for the United Kingdom compared with 53.4 for Japan.

Erosion for Specific Incomes

Tables VI-I and VI-2 show the total erosion of the income on which the income tax is imposed. In Chapter V, it was shown that such erosion affected some types of incomes more than others. It might be appropriate, at this point, to review briefly that evidence.

For France, in 1965 the percentages of the different types of income which were reported were as follows: for wages and salaries, 46.57; for income from real property, 25.65; for income from movable capital, 26.85, and for business income, 23.82.[5]

For Germany, as already indicated, it is only known that 92 per cent of wages and salaries were reported. For the other incomes no data are available, but, as it was argued above, there is indirect evidence to support the belief that the degree of erosion in those other incomes could not have been too high.

For Italy, 33 per cent of wages and salaries were reported in 1962 compared with 27.7 per cent for other incomes.

For the United Kingdom, if reported "actual income"[6] is considered, wages and salaries, in 1962, were about 92 per cent of their counterpart in the national accounts while the other incomes were about 100 per cent. However, if taxable income had been considered, then the percentage for wages and salaries would have decreased somewhat due to reliefs and allowances. The data needed for the change are not available, however.

For Japan, the share of reported wages and salaries in their national income counterpart was about 84 per cent in the last three years while for the other incomes, and especially for agricultural and business incomes, the degree of erosion was much higher.[7]

For the United States, about 87 per cent of wages and salaries as shown by the national accounts are reported but only about 60 per cent of the other incomes.

Tax Evasion

The role that evasion plays in this process of erosion is very difficult to gauge. In Italy and in France, it must be tremendous. In Italy, for example, fiscal evasion is largely condoned by the Church and to a certain extent by the State. There was quite an uproar, some time ago, when the *Osservatore Romano,* the official newspaper of the Vatican, declared in an editorial that tax evasion is not a sin. Such a position may appear paradoxical to anyone not aware of the situation of the common taxpayer in Italy. The Church was simply taking a realistic attitude. In a country where the legal system states that it is no crime to understate one's income up to 25 per cent and where, whether one tells the truth or not, he will not be believed by the authorities, it is naive or unrealistic to expect the average taxpayer to be honest. He knows that regardless of the income he declares, the tax authorities will increase that income considerably, usually by 50 per cent. In fact, by the so-called "analytic" approach, the authority imputes incomes to the tax-

[5] See Table V-4.
[6] See definition in Chapter V, p. 69.
[7] See Table V-15.

payers which often have no relation to those declared and, perhaps, to those received. There follows then a process of bargaining and arguing which may go on for years and which usually benefits the taxpayer by the postponement of his tax payment.

The divergence between incomes declared and those finally ascertained can be seen most glaringly for Italy in the following data for 1962.[8] In that year the number of voluntary declarations was 1,057,000. The tax authorities discovered additional taxpayers numbering more than those who had declared, bringing the total returns to 2,400,000. This discovery, together with the correction of the incomes reported, changed the taxable income from two to three thousand billion lire.

This situation creates a vicious circle whereby the tax authorities attempt to compensate for the substantial evasion by raising the nominal tax rates. Ironically, the very fact that the rates are increased makes tax evasion more profitable.

In Italy, tax evasion is taken for granted and is not denied by either the tax authorities or the general public; Frenchmen, on the other hand, seem to be much more allergic to the accusation of tax cheating. An unpublished study of the French government puts the matter squarely:

> Contrary to a very widespread opinion, fiscal evasion in France is not without any common measure with fiscal evasion in the United States. One forgets very often, in such comparisons, that almost three-fourths of the French taxes are little evaded. One forgets equally the part that vainglory plays in making the French taxpayer boast and the part that puritanism plays in making the American taxpayer hide his fraud.[9]

The evidence on hand, however, strongly contradicts the belief of the French government. Even for the indirect taxes, which constitute the three-fourths of the French taxes which are supposed to be little evaded, some doubts have been raised. Thus, the *Report of the Committee on Turnover Taxation* had this to say on the official control of the value-added tax:

> Taxpaying businesses are visited by inspectors from the tax Administration who conduct an audit to ensure that tax liabilities have been correctly assessed. But the much greater number of businesses to be dealt with imposes upon the tax Administration in France a lower frequency of control visits than under the British purchase tax. We were told that large firms are visited once every three years, medium-sized firms (those with a

[8]The data given are supplied by the Ministry of Finance.

[9]Direction Générale des Impôts, "Comparaison entre les Charges Fiscales Francaises et Américaines" (Paris: no date), p. 7 (my own translation).

turnover exceeding about 40,000 pounds a year) perhaps no more than once in seven or eight years, and smaller firms less frequently still.[10]

The fact that indirect taxes are also evaded to a very high degree is confirmed by a recent study of the Italian General Sales Tax (I.G.E.) in which it is concluded that its evasion may well exceed 50 per cent.[11] A study on tax psychology indicates that 47 per cent of French farmers, 59 per cent of industrialists and businessmen, and 61 per cent of people in liberal professions think that tax evaders are justified.[12]

Another author, after asking whether the "propensity to evade taxes" is higher in some countries than in others, writes that: "In the 'individualistic' Latin countries of the Common Market, for example, tax evasion is knowingly practiced on a much larger scale (30 to 40 per cent) than in their more disciplined Germanic partner-states (10 to 15 per cent). . ."[13] However, he relates that "a recent inquiry in Western Germany[14] found tax morality to be rather low. . ."[15] And he concludes that "it is fair to say that evasion can only occur where evasion opportunities exist."[16]

This last citation is very important and probably much more important than all the statements about tax morality or national propensities for tax evasion. The fact that needs to be emphasized is that Italy and France, in spite of the supposedly high propensity to evade taxes, manage to collect revenues which, in relation to their national income, are among the highest in the western world. It must be assumed, then, that the tax revenues that are lost could not conceivably be recuperated because, if this were done, these two countries would be collecting in revenues perhaps 60 per cent of their gross national product; this is a percentage which, surely, is not conceivable in these types of economies.[17] Therefore, it is a mistake to start with the tax system *as it is* and evaluate fiscal evasion. Such a partial analysis approach is

[10]*Report of the Committee on Turnover Taxation, op. cit.,* pp. 20-21.

[11]Mario Rey, "Estimating Tax Evasions: The Example of the Italian General Sales Tax," *Public Finance,* Vol. XX, Nos. 3-4, 1965, pp. 366-86. Cesare Cosciani has estimated this evasion at 40 per cent. See C. Cosciani, "Tax Reform in Italy: Hopes and Misgivings," *Banca Nazionale del Lavaro Quarterly Review,* September 1967, p. 207.

[12]Jean Duberge, *The Social Psychology of Taxation in France Today* (Paris: 1961), p. 96.

[13]Sylvain Plasschaert, *Taxable Capacity in Developing Countries* (I.B.R.D. and I.D.A., Report No. Ec-103), p. 23.

[14]G. Schmoelders, *Das Irrationale in der Finanzwirtschaft* (Hamburg: 1960).

[15]S. Plasschaert, *op. cit.,* p. 24.

[16]*Ibid.*

[17]It has been reported that the late Luigi Einaudi, former president of Italy and eminent economist, "calculated that, if every tax on the statute books [of Italy] was fully collected, the State would absorb 110 per cent of the national income." See Luigi Barzini, *The Italians* (New York: Bantam Books, Inc., 1965), p. 109.

not admissible in this area. The system of taxation is what it is *because* there is much evasion. It is absurd to assume that it would be the same if taxes were not evaded. For this reason the statement that French and Italians evade 40 per cent of the taxes is really not very meaningful.

The basic issue is not one of tax revenues but one of tax incidence. Which taxes have been made higher by the widespread evasion of the personal income taxes? If the higher taxes are paid by the same people who have been evading the others, then the net effect of evasion would be zero. The answer is that probably all taxes—both income and others—have been made higher, but the net effect has been almost certainly a shift from taxes on income to other forms of taxation which are assumed to be more difficult to evade.

There is an enormous equity problem involved. First, the increase in the legal rates of personal income taxes causes discrimination between those who avoid these taxes and those who find it more difficult to avoid them (mostly recipients of wages and salaries). Second, the increase in so-called indirect taxes usually hurts those who can least afford to pay (though it is impossible to determine this precisely). Taxpayers who have the same ability to pay will have different tastes or different propensities to consume. Indirect taxes will fall harder on those with a low propensity to save and on those whose tastes incline them to purchase the more highly taxed commodities.

TRENDS IN THE PERSONAL INCOME TAX BASES

Table VI-3 provides information on the trend of the erosion of the income tax base for each country. Germany is not shown since no data were available for it. In the table, a better denominator than the gross national product would have been personal income. However, this information is not available for Italy, and, furthermore, its definition is less standardized than that of the gross national product.

The trend of the income tax base was generally upward, while the degree of erosion was being reduced. Of the countries in the table, Japan is the one which shows most progress, increasing the percentage of the gross national product which is reported for personal income taxation from 37.2 to 56.9. If these percentages had been related to personal income rather than to the gross national product, the share would have gone from 49.8 in the former year to 75.8 in the latter year. Coming in the face of a decline in the ratio of the tax to the gross national product, the remarkable increase of the base in Japan is particularly surprising. It is clear that in view of the limited and decreasing erosion, if Japan had wanted to raise substantial revenues from this tax, it could have done so very easily; the fact that it did not must be attributed to a definite policy.

The decrease in erosion for Japan was mostly the result of a larger share of wages and salaries being reported coupled with an increase of the share of national income going to these incomes. In fact, as far as business incomes are concerned, their degree of erosion increased. The same was probably true for incomes from property.

TABLE VI-3. TRENDS IN THE PERSONAL INCOME TAX BASES IN
PERCENTAGES OF GNP, 1955-65.

Years	France	Italy A R.M.	I.C.	United Kingdom A	B	United States A	B	Japan
1955	14.4	17.2	10.9	n.a.	74.5	32.2	57.8	37.2
1956	15.9	19.0	10.7	n.a.	74.1	33.7	59.7	37.1
1957	16.2	21.0	11.3	n.a.	72.8	33.7	59.4	39.1
1958	17.2	21.9	12.1	32.5	71.9	33.6	58.6	42.3
1959	18.0	23.4	13.0	32.9	71.2	34.5	59.5	40.6
1960	16.9	23.3	12.0	35.4	73.5	34.1	58.9	43.8
1961	18.0	24.0	11.2	36.8	75.9	35.0	59.8	45.3
1962	19.1	24.1	11.7	36.2	74.9	35.3	59.1	51.3
1963	21.0	n.a.	n.a.	32.8	71.8	35.5	62.6	53.4
1964	23.0	n.a.	n.a.	n.a.	n.a.	34.3	61.8	56.9
1965	23.4	n.a.	n.a.	n.a.	n.a.	36.8	62.0	n.a.

Notes: A.   Taxable income.
           B.   Reported gross income.
           R.M.   *Ricchezza Mobile.*
           I.C.   *Imposta Complementare.*

Sources: Same as Tables VI-1 and VI-2.

France also shows a substantial reduction in the degree of erosion over the ten-year period; the reported income increased from 14.4 per cent of the gross national product in 1955 to 23 per cent in 1964. If the effective average tax rate on reported income had remained the same over the period, the ratio of the tax to the gross national product would have increased much more than it did in view of the reduction in the erosion. In France, however, in the same way as in Japan, the reduction in tax rates compensated for the relative increase in reported income. Thus, increasing revenues were obtained in spite of a decrease in the effective average tax rate on reported income.

In the previous chapter, it was pointed out that in France the degree of erosion was reduced in all of the major income categories with especially notable gains in income from real property for which the reported share increased from 7.8 in 1955 to 32 in 1964. For wages and salaries the share increased from 28.26 to 44.51; for incomes from movable capital the increase was from 17.33 to 29.06; for incomes from business, the gain was the smallest—from 15.11 to 23.26.

Italy showed some progress in the reduction of the erosion over the decade. But it was mostly limited to the *Ricchezza Mobile,* the base of which in relation to the gross national product increased from 17.2 to 24.1. The *Im-*

posta Complementare, on the other hand, did not show much of an increase and the degree of erosion remained extremely high.[18]

Table V-10 showed that for the four schedules of the *Ricchezza Mobile,* A and B show increasing effective average tax rates on reported income, while C_1 and C_2 show either constant or decreasing ones. For the four schedules combined, the effective average tax rate on reported income decreased from 10.3 in 1954-55 to 9.7 in 1962. For the *Imposta Complementare,* the effective average tax rate increased from 2.6 to 3.3; however, the revenues from this tax account for only a small share of the total revenues. Thus, the increase in the T/GNP ratio that took place during the period can be attributed mainly to the reduction in the erosion of the *Ricchezza Mobile* and to a much smaller degree to the increase in the effective rate for the *Imposta Complementare.*

The experience of the United Kingdom was quite different from that of the three countries previously discussed. In fact, not much change in the degree of erosion took place. If the two extreme years are considered, the degree of erosion with respect to reported income increased with the ratio of reported income to personal income decreasing from 74.5 in 1955 to 71.8 in 1963. This fact, is particularly relevant since it was accompanied by a substantial increase in the T/GNP ratio. Thus, this increase could be attributed only to an increase in the effective average tax rate on reported income.

For the United States, the degree of erosion appears to have decreased over the period from about 32.2 per cent to 35.5 per cent with respect to taxable income. The decrease resulted in increasing the T/GNP ratio without any increase in the effective average tax rate on taxable income.

The reduction in the degrees of erosion which has been discussed above was reflected, at least in part, in the increase in the number of tax returns. The increases, all expressed in thousands, were as follows: in France from 4,401 in 1957 to 7,725 in 1964; in Italy from 4,077 in 1955 to 4,242 in 1963; in the United Kingdom from 20,100 in 1955 to 21,925 in 1964; in Japan from 10,969 in 1955 to 19,242 in 1964, and in the United States from 44,689 in 1955 to 51,323 in 1963. For Germany, the constitutional reform concerning income splitting decreased the number of tax returns from 20,512 in 1957 to 15,581 in 1958. Since 1958, however, the number has been increasing; in 1961, for the wage tax the returns were 20,670.

EROSION AS A DETERMINANT OF THE DIFFERENCES IN INCOME TAX BURDENS

Table IV-6 above provided several definitions of income tax burden. According to the first column of that table the tax burdens for the six countries

[18]The revenues from this tax have increased substantially since 1963; thus, perhaps, the trend shown in the table may have been reversed.

were quite different. The question that may be raised at this point is: What part of those differences could be attributed to differences in erosion? In other words, what would the burden be if, for example, all the countries had the same degree of erosion as the United States? This is, of course, a completely hypothetical question. In making the adjustments, it will be assumed that the changes in the base implied by the correctional coefficients bear the same average tax rate as the actual bases.

The correctional coefficients are obtained by dividing the United States base by that of each other country. The coefficients thus obtained are: 1.69 for France; 1.47 for Italy; .98 for the United Kingdom; 1.17 for Japan. When these coefficients are multiplied by the burdens of Table IV-6, the hypothetical burdens are obtained. Table VI-4 gives both actual and hypothetical burdens. It shows what differences in the burdens by country can be attributed to the rate structure rather than to differences in relative bases. In other words, a correction of the difference in coverage would still leave differences which can be attributed exclusively to the effective average tax rates. A correction of the bases to the level of that of the United States would increase the burdens for France, Italy, and Japan, but would still leave their burdens much behind those of the United States and the United Kingdom.

TABLE VI-4. ACTUAL AND HYPOTHETICAL TAX BURDENS, 1963

Countries	Actual	Hypothetical
France	3.1	5.2
Germany	9.0	n.a.
Italy	4.2	6.2
Japan	4.2	4.9
United Kingdom	9.9	9.7
United States	10.2	10.2

Source: Table IV-6 and text.

CONCLUSIONS

This chapter has dealt with the various aspects of the erosion to which the income tax systems of all the countries are inevitably subjected. The objective was to show how important income tax erosion is in the determination of the ratio of the personal income tax revenues to the gross national product. Whenever taxable income was not available, an indication of erosion was the divergence of reported income from the gross national product.

The estimates obtained show that—of the five countries for which the information was available—the United States and the United Kingdom are the two with the smallest degree of erosion; France and Italy are the two with the highest degree. Japan is in-between, but closer to the former.

Tax evasion is, of course, one of the important determinants of erosion. The information available on this aspect of erosion is limited but it is sufficient to indicate that in France and Italy it is very high and much higher than in the other countries. It is, however, argued that contrary to a common belief, this is probably more the consequence of greater opportunities for tax evasion than the reflection of national backgrounds, although the latter element does play a role.

The chapter also analyzes some dynamic aspects of erosion in order to see whether it was decreasing or increasing over the period. Most countries show some increases in the ratio of the tax base to the gross national product. Of these Japan was by far the one with the greatest success, increasing that ratio from 37.2 in 1955 to 56.9 in 1964 (these ratios refer to reported income rather than to taxable income).

Japan's remarkable progress was undoubtedly in part the reflection of the Japanese industrial development of the period. As a country becomes industrialized, more and more of its national income originates in activities for which tax control is easier; or, it is received in forms—such as wages and salaries—which don't lend themselves to income tax evasion. Thus, during such a process, if the country is willing, it can easily increase the revenues of this tax, even if it maintains the same average effective tax rate on taxable or reported income. There is a limit, however, to this possibility. Once the degree of evasion is reduced to the level of, say, that of the United States and the United Kingdom then this possibility becomes much more limited, although, as the studies by Pechman, Goode, and others have shown, there is still some ground for improvement in this direction. At this level of erosion, relative increases in the revenues from the personal income tax are more dependent on increases in rates than on broadening of the base.

France and, to a lesser extent, Italy have also succeeded in decreasing their degree of erosion although not as much as Japan. The difference between these two countries and Japan is that while the latter compensated for the broadening of the base by cutting the rates and increasing the size of the exemptions, the former did not, so that the reduction in erosion was in part reflected in relative increases in tax revenues.

For the United Kingdom, the experience was somewhat different from that of the other three countries since erosion increased during the period but it was more than compensated by an increase in the effective average tax rate on taxable income. In the United States, on the other hand, the increase in the tax burden was due to both an increase in the effective average tax rate on adjusted gross income and a reduction in erosion.

VII

DYNAMIC ASPECTS OF THE
INDIVIDUAL INCOME TAXES

Up to now this study has been concerned mainly with static aspects of the individual income taxes in the countries considered. Although, at times, the analysis has covered more than just one year, the reference to several years has been only incidental. I shall now look at the dynamic or historical relationships between the revenues from the tax and the national income in each country.

FRANCE

General Characteristics

The limited importance of the French personal income tax as well as its rather erratic character is seen clearly in Table VII-1, which also shows the behavior of the tax in relation to the gross national product for the 1950-65 period. The ratio of the tax to the gross national product has fluctuated between 2 and 3 per cent for most of the years, coming closer to the latter figure recently and exceeding it in 1964 and 1965. The variation is so small that it is not worthwhile to trace the various tax cuts which have been enacted over the period.

Several times over the period under consideration the French tax authorities have increased the size of the brackets to which the nominal rates (which with minor modifications have remained the same) apply. Thus, the conscious fiscal legislation was aimed at decreasing the revenues from this tax. However, there have been two major forces which have caused the increase in revenues from the tax to exceed the increase of the gross national product. The first is the increase in per capita income which has moved the taxpayers toward higher nominal rates; the second is the progressive lowering of the erosion. The net effect of these two factors has been a general increase in the ratio of the tax to the gross national product. Basically, in the absence of tax cuts, the elasticity of the tax was substantially greater than one.

89

TABLE VII-1. RELATIONSHIP BETWEEN PERSONAL INCOME TAX AND GNP
FOR FRANCE, 1950-65

(francs in billions)

Years	Personal income taxes[a] (T)	GNP	$\frac{T}{GNP}$	$\frac{\triangle T}{\triangle GNP}$	$\frac{\triangle T/T}{\triangle GNP/GNP}$
1950	2.10	100.20	2.09%	—	—
1951	2.38	122.90	1.94	1.23%	0.59%
1952	3.04	144.04	2.11	3.13	1.61
1953	3.95	151.91	2.60	11.56	5.48
1954	3.65	160.81	2.27	−3.37	−1.30
1955	3.41	170.50	2.00	−2.48	−0.93
1956	4.32	188.32	2.23	5.11	2.54
1957	5.04	211.11	2.39	4.04	1.38
1958	6.36	244.71	2.60	3.93	1.65
1959	7.97	267.38	2.98	7.10	2.72
1960	7.89	296.22	2.66	−0.28	−0.09
1961	8.47	319.69	2.65	2.47	0.94
1962	9.75	356.29	2.74	3.50	1.32
1963	11.44	395.58	2.89	4.30	1.56
1964	14.23	431.87	3.29	7.69	2.65
1965	15.91	461.44	3.45	5.68	1.74

[a]Includes both the progressive and the complementary tax.

Source: France, Ministère de L'Economie et des Finances, *Statistiques et Etudes Financière,* Supplement (Paris: Imprimerie Nationale, many years); O.E.C.D. *National Accounts Statistics* (Paris: O.E.C.D.)

The reform of 1959 had an important effect on revenues as shown in the table. Most of the rise in tax revenues which followed that reform is due to the increasing participation of wages and salaries in the total.[1] Since the share of wages and salaries in the national income was increasing, the income tax was, in Dosser's terminology, dynamic progressive.[2]

The revenues from the tax for 1963 (F11.44 billion) amounted to only 15.4 per cent of the government's transfers to the families (74.22 billion francs[3]). This clearly shows what a limited role the French income tax plays in the redistribution of income in France.

Cyclical Behavior

Another interesting aspect of the French personal income tax is its performance during the business cycle. Although the revenue from this tax has shown some tendency to increase it has behaved perversely during periods of slow-down in the French economy. There were two such "recessions" in

[1]See Table V-3, p. 57.

[2]D. Dosser, "Tax Incidence and Growth," *The Economic Journal,* Vol. LXXI, September 1961.

[3]E.E.C. *General Statistical Bulletin,* No. 11, 1964, p. 85.

France: one in 1953, and the other in 1959, and there was also a slow-down in 1961. By "recession" here is meant a deviation from the trend rather than an actual decline in the gross national product. The gross national product continued to rise in these periods although at a slower rate.

The table shows that it was during these years of recession that the tax was most productive. In fact, as a percentage of the gross national product, it jumped from 2.11 in 1952 to 2.60 in 1953 to decline again during the high growth years between 1953 and 1957 (when the gross national product at constant prices increased at a rate of over 5 per cent) to barely over 2 per cent. In 1958-59 when the rate of growth of the gross national product fell considerably—to around 2 per cent—the same reaction took place. During the most serious recession year—1959—the ratio of the tax to the gross national product reached the highest level of any year except 1964 and 1965. The ratio declined again in the upswing of 1960 only to increase during the slowdown of 1961.

The flexibility of the tax was such that in the recession years the $\triangle T/\triangle GNP$ ratio became quite high (11.56 in 1953 and 7.1 in 1959) while in the years succeeding a recession it became negative. Such perverse reaction of the income tax to the cycle is a consequence of the collection method since the taxes are collected on the year after the incomes have been earned. Thus, if a boom year is succeeded by a recession year, people will be paying the taxes due on the incomes earned in the boom year during the recession.

GERMANY

General Characteristics

Germany is a classical case in which fiscal policy has been geared almost exclusively to growth. Such a redirection has been so extreme that it has often been accused of being antisocial.

The dynamism of the German fiscal policy, as applied to growth, is reflected by the frequent changes, at least up to 1958, in the income tax legislation. These changes transformed this tax, in the relatively short span of a decade, from probably the most progressive personal income tax in the world to one of the least. Progressivity as a means of redistributing income was all but given up and other measures were substituted for it. The main result of these changes was that 95 per cent of all taxpayers and 98 per cent of all wage earners were excluded from progression and that more than half of all persons gainfully employed were not subject to income taxation.[4] These changes are reflected in glaring fashion by Table VII-2.

[4]Henry J. Grunpel and Carl Boettcher, *Taxation in the Federal Republic of Germany* ("World Tax Series"; Cambridge, Mass.: Harvard Law School, 1963), p. 138.

TABLE VII-2. BASIC EXEMPTION AND HIGHEST MARGINAL RATES OF
INDIVIDUAL INCOME TAXES IN GERMANY

(DM)

Period	Income free of taxes (Basic exemption)	Highest marginal rate (HMR)	Income at which HMR applies
1946-June 1948	600	95.00%	60,000
July 1948-1949	750	95.00	250,000
1950	750	95.00	250,000
1951-1952	750	95.00	250,000
1953	750	82.25	220,000
1954	800	80.00	220,000
1955-1957	900	63.45	605,001
since 1958	1700	53.00	110,040

Source: Karl Häuser, "West Germany," N.B.E.R. and The Brookings Institution,
Foreign Tax Policies and Economic Growth (Washington, D.C.: The Brookings Institution, 1966), p. 147.

The table shows that the size of the basic exemption which, in the immediate after-war period, was DM600 was progressively increased to the level of DM1,710. At the same time the highest marginal rate was lowered from a peak of 95 per cent which, for some incomes from property because of the existence of wealth tax could amount to more than 100 per cent, to its present and comparatively mild level of 53 per cent.

Of interest, also, is the level of income at which the *total* tax paid is 50 per cent of the taxable income (i.e. the average tax rate is 50 per cent). This information is provided below.

Table VII-3 confirms that the personal income tax on high income groups in Germany has become gradually much lighter. During the postwar period an income of only DM14,200 would hit an average rate of 50 per cent; by 1958 it would take an income almost 27 times higher (DM376,033) to reach the same average rate.

TABLE VII-3. INCOMES WITH AVERAGE TAX RATES OF 50 PER CENT

(DM)

Period	Income
1946-June 1948	14,200
July 1948-1949	25,000
1950	61,500
1951-1952	61,500
1953	82,800
1954	110,000
1955-57	341,000
since 1958	376,033

Source: Same as in Table VII-2.

Cyclical Behavior

The net result of these reforms has been to change the burden of the tax and has affected the elasticity and the flexibility of the personal income tax. Analytical attempts at measuring the elasticity and flexibility of a certain nominal structure of the personal income tax are interesting only when the tax laws remain unchanged for a considerable length of time as has generally been the case in the United States. However, due to the dynamism of the German legislation in the fiscal field,[5] only ex-post calculations have meaning. Table VII-4 reports the computation of the elasticity and the flexibility of the combined personal income taxes together with the annual ratios of their revenue to the gross national product of Germany.

TABLE VII-4. RELATIONSHIP BETWEEN PERSONAL INCOME TAXES
AND GNP FOR GERMANY, 1950-65

(DM in billions)

Years	Combined personal income taxes (T)	GNP	$\frac{T}{GNP}$	$\frac{\Delta T}{\Delta GNP}$	$\frac{\Delta T/T}{\Delta GNP/GNP}$
1950	3.9	97.8	4.03%	–	–
1951	5.2	118.6	4.37	5.87%	1.46%
1952	7.7	135.6	5.67	14.76	3.38
1953	8.8	147.1	5.95	9.30	1.64
1954	8.7	157.9	5.52	−0.09	−0.07
1955	9.1	180.4	5.04	1.64	0.30
1956	10.5	198.8	5.30	7.88	1.57
1957	11.6	216.3	5.38	6.28	1.18
1958	11.9	231.5	5.14	1.71	0.33
1959	14.0	250.9	5.58	10.77	2.10
1960	17.9	296.8	6.03	8.49	1.52
1961	22.3	326.2	6.82	14.76	2.44
1962	25.7	354.5	7.23	12.04	1.76
1963	28.4	377.6	7.55	12.59	1.50
1964	31.4	413.8	7.58	8.29	1.10
1965	32.9	448.8	7.33	4.29	0.57

Source: Germany, Deutsche Bundesbank, *Monthly Report* (Frankfurt).

From the table it can be realized that almost every year

$$\frac{\Delta T_1}{\Delta GNP_1} > \frac{T_0}{GNP_0}$$

which implies that the combined revenue, at least in an ex-post sense, was quite elastic. The effects of the tax reforms of 1954-55, 1958, and 1964 are

[5]O. Buehler has estimated that in the period 1951-56 an average of 615 sections of tax laws were amended annually. Reported in Frederick G. Reuss, *Fiscal Policy for Growth without Inflation* (Baltimore: The Johns Hopkins Press, 1963), p. 39.

clearly reflected in both the flexibility and the elasticity of the tax. It is quite obvious, however, that, apart from these temporary halts, the German personal income tax has had an elasticity of well over one. This elasticity accounts for the considerable automatic increase in the ratio of the tax to the gross national product whenever there is no reform to prevent it. From 1958 to 1963, the ratio of the tax to the gross national product increased from 5.14 to 7.55. In 1958, 45 per cent of the residents of Germany were not subject to income tax due to their limited earnings. By 1963, this percentage had been reduced to 25 per cent. Such an increase is quite drastic and is bound to affect personal saving.[6]

This possibility has been a major factor in inducing the German government to try to alleviate the weight of the tax. On April 14, 1964 a bill was introduced for this purpose. The bill was approved by the German parliament and became effective on January 1, 1965. The new income tax law has alleviated the burden of personal income tax on the middle class. An attempt at increasing the size of the basic exemption was rejected.[7]

Table VII-4 indicates that for the period 1960-64, during which there was no major reform in the income tax legislation, the built-in flexibility of the combined revenues of the income taxes was around 12 per cent, while the elasticity was above 1.5. For the specific income taxes the built-in flexibility was around 6 per cent for the wage tax, around 5 per cent for the assessed tax, and around 1 per cent for the capital yield tax.[8] These estimates have been obtained from the data in Table VII-5 where the actual elasticities of the specific income taxes have been calculated. These elasticities appear to be substantially higher than one, especially for the wage tax.

No estimates are available regarding the built-in flexibility of German income taxes during a recession. In view of the frequent changes in the tax structure, it would be very difficult to obtain those estimates. Such estimates would necessarily have to evaluate the collection method of each of the three income taxes. Of these, only the wage tax, being withheld at the source, accompanies the fluctuation of income and thus it would offer prospects for anticyclical behavior. The other two taxes are paid with considerable lags, and, when they are anticipated—as for the assessed tax, they are paid on the basis of the income of the previous year and thus they may accentuate rather than smooth the cycle.

[6]See Chapter V, pp. 63-64.

[7]International Bureau of Fiscal Documentation, *European Taxation,* March 1965, pp. 64-65; see also Chapter II above.

[8]For the period 1955-60, Paul Senf reports somewhat lower estimates. His estimates are 2.31 for the wage tax and 2.47 for the assessed tax. See his comment on Karl Häuser, "West Germany," N.B.E.R. and The Brookings Institution, *Foreign Tax Policies and Economic Growth* (New York: Columbia University Press, 1966), p. 162.

TABLE VII-5. ELASTICITIES OF THE THREE PERSONAL INCOME TAXES
IN GERMANY, 1950-65

(DM in millions)

Years	Wage tax	Assessed income tax	Capital yield tax	GNP (billions)	Elasticities		
					Wage tax	Assessed income tax	Capital yield tax
1950	1,806.5	2,087.4	31.8	97.8	–	–	–
1951	2,796.5	2,302.7	84.0	118.6	2.57%	0.48%	7.70%
1952	3,658.1	3,925.4	111.2	135.6	2.15	4.90	2.26
1953	3,740.4	4,870.4	151.8	147.1	0.26	2.83	4.29
1954	3,874.5	4,587.9	259.7	157.9	0.49	−0.84	9.73
1955	4,402.1	4,351.7	341.3	180.4	0.96	−0.38	2.21
1956	5,402.1	4,728.0	417.8	198.8	1.23	0.84	2.20
1957	5,289,0	5,879.2	481.3	216.3	−0.24	2.76	1.73
1958	5,932.3	5,473.3	509.3	231.5	1.74	−1.06	0.83
1959	5,855.3	7,323.2	829.7	250.9	−0.15	4.02	7.49
1960	8,101.7	8,963.3	846.1	296.8	2.10	1.22	0.11
1961	10,453.1	10,817.4	980.1	326.2	2.93	2.09	1.60
1962	12,314.9	12,218.3	1,130.3	354.5	2.05	1.49	1.76
1963	13,844.4	13,451.2	1,137.8	377.6	1.91	1.54	0.10
1964	16,092.1	14,100.9	1,252.3	413.8	1.69	0.50	1.05
1965	16,738.0	14,798.4	1,350.7	448.8	0.47	0.59	0.92

Source: Same as Table VII-4.

ITALY

General Characteristics

The relative importance of the personal income tax in Italy is comparable
to that of France; the Italian tax, however, shows much stabler features than
the French. From Table VII-6, it can be seen that it has increased continuously from 210.4 billion lire in 1952 to 1,268.6 billion lire in 1965. As a
share of the gross national product, it has increased every single year from
1.86 per cent in 1952 to 3.58 per cent in 1965.[9]

Such an increase was the result of an elasticity greater than one. In fact, in
most of the years considered, such elasticity was substantially greater than
one as shown in the last column of the table. Because of the very limited
progressivity of the income taxes in Italy, this elasticity must be attributed
mainly to changes in the tax base. It must be recalled that the revenues from
schedule B of the *Ricchezza Mobile* are mostly from the income of corporations, while those of schedule C_2 are from incomes from wages and salaries.
The development of the Italian economy, by increasing the profits of the
business enterprises and the share of wages and salaries in the national income, has substantially increased the base on which the *Ricchezza Mobile* is
imposed.

[9] These estimates include the revenues from schedule B of the *Ricchezza Mobile*.

TABLE VII-6. RELATIONSHIP BETWEEN PERSONAL INCOME TAXES
AND GNP FOR ITALY, 1952-65

(lire in billions)

Years	Personal income taxes[a]	GNP	$\frac{T}{GNP}$	$\frac{\Delta T}{\Delta GNP}$	$\frac{\Delta T/T}{\Delta GNP/GNP}$
1952	210.4	11,289	1.86%	–	–
1953	241.5	12,486	1.93	2.60%	1.39%
1954	281.3	13,324	2.11	4.75	2.45
1955	325.2	14,641	2.22	3.33	1.58
1956	382.7	15,908	2.41	4.54	2.03
1957	421.9	17,081	2.47	3.34	1.38
1958	482.6	18,340	2.63	4.82	1.95
1959	522.8	19,437	2.69	3.66	1.39
1960	590.6	21,071	2.80	4.15	1.55
1961	681.9	23,363	2.92	3.98	1.42
1962	794.8	26,330	3.02	3.81	1.30
1963	939.1	30,193	3.11	3.74	1.24
1964	1.161.2[b]	33,112	3.53	7.91	2.46
1965	1.268.6[b]	35,460	3.58	4.57	1.31

[a]For fiscal years.

[b]Calendar years.

Sources: Italy, Ministero delle Finanze, *L'Attività Tributaria dal 1954 al 1964*
(Rome: Istituto Poligrafico dello Stato, 1964) Vol. I; Ministero delle Finance, *L'Attivitá
Tributaria nel 1965* (Rome: Istituto Poligrafico dello Stato, 1966); O.E.C.D., *National
Accounts Statistics* (Paris: O.E.C.D.).

Because of its relatively small magnitude, the impact of the personal income tax on the Italian economy is obviously small. This is particularly true
if schedule B is considered separately. Similarly, its redistributive power is as
limited as that of France. However, it must be realized (and this is also true
for France) that some people may pay substantial income taxes, since in
relation to the income tax *base* the income tax payments have averaged
around 10 per cent in both Italy and France.

Cyclical Behavior

The elastic character of the tax in the upswing makes the flexibility greater
than the ratio of the tax to the gross national product. Table VII-6 shows the
estimates for the flexibility average around 4 per cent—too small to be of any
consequence. I have tried to analyze the reaction of the tax to the cyclical
changes in the gross national product. To do so, I have evaluated the yearly
percentage changes in the ratio of the tax to the gross national product, and I
have related these percentages to the yearly percentage changes in the gross
national product at constant prices. The results are shown graphically in
Figure VII-1. It is quite evident that in Italy, though not in the same way as
in France, the relationship is an inverse one. In other words, the higher was

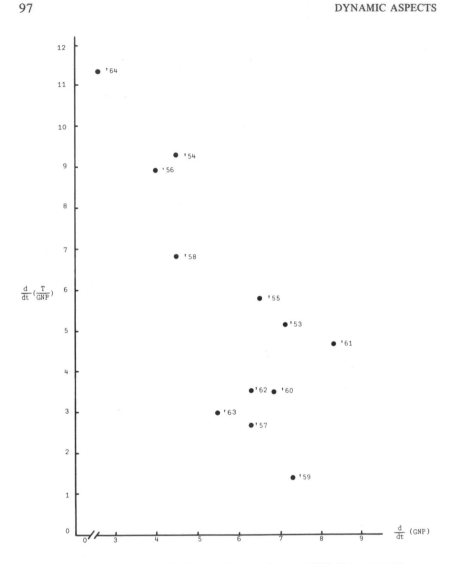

Figure VII-1. Relationship Between Income Tax and GNP, Italy, 1954-64.

the rate of change of the gross national product the lower was the rate of change of the ratio of the tax to the gross national product.

Although, as it has been seen above, the elasticity of the income taxes has been positive with respect to upward movements in the gross national product, it is doubtful if the tax would help to prevent a fall in the national income. Apart from its limited scope, the basic limitation is the method of assessment and collection which seems to introduce a systematic lag between changes in the national income and changes in tax revenues.

The taxpayer normally reports this year's income on the basis of last year's results. Furthermore, the tax authorities publish the tax rolls around June and the agencies in charge start collecting at the end of the year or at the beginning of the next; the collection may go on for the first half of the next year. Therefore, there may be a lag of up to one and a half years from the time the income is earned to the time the tax is paid. Even when the tax is withheld at the source, as in the case of some wages, the lag still persists since, although the withholding on the part of the enterprises is contemporaneous with the earning of income, the remittance to the tax authorities of the amounts withheld does not take place at the same time. Instead, the enterprises are required by law to pay during the current year, in six separate installments, the equivalent of the taxes that the wage earner paid the previous year. It is clear that whenever wages are increasing the enterprises will withhold more than they have to transfer immediately to the authorities. The enterprise is required to pay the balance due the following August.

Because of the previous reasons, it is easy to see that the income taxes of Italy cannot in any way be relied upon for providing some built-in flexibility in business cycles.

JAPAN

General Characteristics

Of the countries which have been considered in this study, Japan has the highest rate of growth. The gross national product of this country has been increasing at exceptional rates. In view of this, it is interesting to analyze the reaction of the Japanese income tax to the growth of the gross national product.

The base of the personal income tax—i.e., the share of the personal income which has been subjected to taxation—has been quite high in Japan, and, furthermore, it has been increasing. In view of this, and in spite of the relatively low nominal rates, the tax has been very elastic with respect to the gross national product. This elasticity has averaged well over two for the period considered—not only the consequence of progressivity of the nominal rates but also of increase in the base.

In view of this situation, if the tax authorities of Japan had remained passive, the share of the personal income tax in the gross national product would have increased to levels not desired by the Japanese authorities and which would have been damaging to the growth of the economy. In other words, given the public expenditure of Japan, the government would have been faced with very embarassing surpluses, which would have inevitably put a drag on growth.

The answer to this situation was formalized in a "tax-cut policy" which consisted in the annual reduction of the nominal rates and or the annual increase of the basic exemptions. The rationale for this policy was very similar to that which led to the 1964 tax cut in the United States. The results of this policy can be seen in the tables. Table VII-7 shows what the tax burden would have been, in the absence of the tax reductions, as compared to the actual tax burden. The hypothetical tax burden is calculated with the assumption that the growth of the gross national product would have been the same; this, however, is hardly a realistic assumption in view of the extremely high level which would have been reached by the tax burden: 55.2 in 1963! Table VII-7 concerns all the tax revenues rather than just the income tax but most of the increase can be safely attributed to this tax because of its elasticity and importance.

TABLE VII-7. ESTIMATES OF JAPANESE TAX REVENUE AND
TAX BURDEN IN THE ABSENCE OF TAX REFORMS AFTER 1950

(yen in billions)

Fiscal year	National income (A)		Tax Revenue				Tax burden	
			Settled amounts (B)	Tax reduction (C)	Estimates without reform (D)		$\frac{(B)}{(A)}$	$\frac{(D)}{(A)}$
1949	(100)	2,737	518	—	(100)	518	18.9%	18.7%
1950	(124)	3,382	338	213	(106)	551	10.0	16.3
1951	(165)	4,525	551	413	(186)	964	12.2	21.3
1952	(186)	5,085	716	658	(265)	1,375	14.1	27.0
1953	(210)	5,748	761	1,037	(347)	1,789	13.2	31.3
1954	(220)	6,022	776	1,135	(369)	1,911	12.9	31.7
1955	(245)	6,719	788	1,271	(397)	2,059	11.7	30.6
1956	(279)	7,628	971	1,462	(469)	2,432	12.7	31.9
1957	(303)	8,286	1,085	1,705	(539)	2,790	13.1	33.7
1958	(311)	8,519	1,053	1,851	(561)	2,904	12.4	34.1
1959	(367)	10,037	1,252	2,365	(698)	3,617	12.5	36.0
1960	(435)	11,904	1,468	3,216	(904)	4,684	12.3	39.3
1961	(516)	14,118	2,048	4,003	(1,168)	6,051	14.5	42.9
1962	(560)	15,320	2,225	5,070	(1,408)	7,295	14.5	47.6
1963	(608)	16,650	2,341	6,845	(1,773)	9,187	14.1	55.2

Note: GNP elasticity of Tax Revenue = 1.75.

Source: This table was obtained from the statistical appendix to Ryutaro Komiya, "Taxation and Capital Formation in Postwar Japan." This study was revised and published without the appendix as "Japan" in N.B.E.R. and The Brookings Institution, *Foreign Tax Policies and Economic Growth* (New York: Columbia University Press, 1966).

Table VII-8 shows the minimum taxable income for wage earners in several family situations for the period 1950-64. It can be seen that in 1964 the minimum taxable income was at least five times the level of 1950 and that

TABLE VII-8. CHANGES IN THE LEVELS OF NONTAXABLE INCOME
FOR WAGE EARNERS IN JAPAN, 1950-66

(yen)

Years	Single	Number of dependents			
		1 (Spouse)	2	3	4
1950	29,412	43,350	57,648	71,765	85,883
1951	44,784	64,706	84,706	104,706	122,353
1952	61,350	85,890	109,757	134,147	152,440
1953	73,620	115,854	140,244	164,635	182,927
1954	83,841	131,251	160,638	190,024	207,750
1955	93,540	143,124	174,238	205,071	223,714
1956	100,000	150,000	181,250	212,500	231,250
1957	115,588	178,336	210,776	243,710	263,470
1958	118,781	184,770	217,220	250,132	269,879
1959	118,781	204,055	241,904	279,753	313,156
1960	118,781	210,638	250,132	289,627	327,912
1961	129,338	247,498	286,992	325,287	390,870
1962	139,236	267,245	305,613	344,962	408,916
1963	151,894	288,335	322,720	377,104	438,632
1964	172,935	316,017	367,043	417,614	471,377
1965	196,607	351,130	413,163	474,036	544,245
1966	220,278	387,953	463,084	537,282	613,421

Note: Minimum taxable income is computed by adding the basic exemption, exemptions for spouse and dependents, employment income deduction and social insurance premium deduction.

Source: Japan, Ministry of Finance, Tax Bureau, *An Outline of Japanese Taxes* (Tokyo: annual).

practically every year the size of the minimum taxable income was increased. These increases, together with the lowering of the rates, substantially reduced the average income tax rate on all the income levels. For example, on incomes of 500 thousand yen, the rate fell from 32.7 in 1950 to 12.93 in 1955 to 3.28 in 1960 and to .74 in 1964. For incomes of 1 million yen, the rates for the same years were 43.33, 26.21, 11.11, and 6.56. For incomes of 5 million yen they were 52.66, 49.48, 31.51, and 29.38. Finally, for incomes of 10 million yen the rates were 53.83, 57.12, 40.10, and 39.05. In view of the substantial increases in personal exemptions, the reduction in the average rates was more significant at the low levels than at the higher levels.[10]

The increase in the size of the exemptions had also the effect of decreasing, for most kinds of income, the proportion of income earners who were subjected to the personal income tax. For agricultural income this proportion was reduced from 38.1 per cent in 1950 to 6.2 per cent in 1962; for non-agricultural business income the reduction was from 49.7 per cent to 22.7 per

[10]This information is taken from the appendix to Ryutaro Komiya, "Taxation and Capital Formation in Postwar Japan." This study was revised and published without the appendix as "Japan" in *Forcign Tax Policies, op. cit.*

cent; for employment income, it was from 78.5 per cent to 59.5 per cent. The effect of these changes was to increase the proportion of the employment-income earners from 69.6 per cent in 1950 to 86.5 per cent in 1962.

Table VII-9 gives a breakdown of the relative contributions of the basic exemption, exemption for dependents, rates and others in the total annual reductions. Individually, the rate reductions were the most important followed closely by the reductions in the basic exemption and in the exemptions for dependents. Combined, however, the latter two were more important than the rate reductions.

Cyclical Behavior

Table VII-10 gives the main relationships between the personal income tax and the gross national product for a period of twelve years. The first column provides the actual revenues from the income tax in each year. The fourth column gives the estimates of the revenues from the income tax which would have been obtained in a year t on the basis of the tax legislation which prevailed in the year t-1. In other words these estimates have been obtained by adding to the actual revenues the amount of the annual total tax reductions given in Table VII-9. The estimates of the flexibility have been calculated by subtracting from the estimate for the tax revenue without reform in a given year t (column 4) the actual revenue from the previous year t-1, (column 1) and dividing that difference by the gross national product. It was necessary to follow this method because, otherwise, in view of the sizeable yearly cuts, the estimates would have been meaningless. The same approach was followed for the calculations of the elasticities in the last column.

The burden of the tax over the years shown has followed two different trends: from 1953 to 1959 it declined consistently from 4.1 to 2.2; from 1959 onward it increased—also consistently—reaching a height of 3.3 in 1964. During this period there was one recession (1958) and two slow-downs (1960 and 1962).

It is interesting to observe the flexibility and elasticity of the tax for those years. In 1958, which witnessed a full-fledged recession, the estimate of the flexibility (keeping in mind how it was calculated) was 5.6 while that of the elasticity was 2.27. In 1960 the corresponding estimates were 5.4 and 2.43 while in 1962 they were 9.8 and 3.5. These are relatively high values; in fact, on the average, they are higher than for most of the other years. It is interesting to observe now the estimates of the flexibility and the elasticity for the years 1959, 1961, and 1963, which were periods of high prosperity. In these years the estimates of the flexibility and more particularly of the elasticity are quite low: the elasticity went down from 2.27 in 1958 to .77 in 1959; from 2.43 in 1960 to 1.98 in 1961; and from 3.5 in 1962 to 1.73 in 1963.

TABLE VII-9. AMOUNTS OF INCOME TAX REDUCTION BY TAX
REFORM, 1950-66

(yen in million)

	1950	1951	1952	1953	1954	1955	1956	1957	1958	1959	1960	1961	1962	1963	1964	1965	1966
Exemptions and Deductions:																	
Basic	324	186	575	239	179	157	—	201	—	—	—	—	161	180	222	229	259
Dependents	611	244	245	267	102	—	—	129	—	278	—	204	77	134	180	412	267
Employment Income	+212	—	—	95	—	57	226	70	—	—	—	102	—	—	226	225	409
Others	9	30	121	—	7	91	—	+53	—	—	—	75	43	6	109	56	108
Sub Total	732	460	941	601	288	305	226	347	—	278	—	381	281	320	737	922	1,044
Rates	411	147	210	92	—	132	—	854	—	123	—	234	430	—	—	—	533
Total	1,143	607	1,151	693	288	438	226	1,201	—	401	—	615	711	320	737	922	1,577
Others	215	+2	+24	80	26	96	—	+99	63	+170	—	+52	+10	348	8	268	6
Total	1,358	605	1,127	773	314	533	226	1,102	63	231	—	563	701	668	745	654	1,583

Note: The amount of tax reduction is the amount of reduction in the normal year computed on the basis of anticipated revenues for each fiscal year.

Source: Japan, Ministry of Finance, Tax Bureau, *An Outline of Japanese Taxes* (Tokyo: annual).

TABLE VII-10. RELATIONSHIP OF PERSONAL INCOME TAX REVENUES
TO GNP FOR JAPAN, 1953-64

(yen in billions)

Years	Personal income tax (1)	GNP (2)	$\frac{T}{GNP}$ (3)	Tax without Reform (4)	$\frac{\Delta T}{\Delta GNP}$ (5)	$\frac{\Delta T/T}{\Delta GNP/GNP}$ (6)
1953	292.5	7,084.8	4.1%	369.6	–	–
1954	285.6	7,465.7	3.8	317.0	6.4%	1.56%
1955	278.7	8,235.5	3.4	332.0	6.0	1.58
1956	304.9	9,292.9	3.3	327.5	4.6	1.36
1957	251.8	10,149.8	2.5	362.0	6.7	2.03
1958	259.3	10,394.7	2.5	265.6	5.6	2.27
1959	278.0	12,572.5	2.2	301.1	1.9	0.77
1960	390.6	14,671.4	2.7	390.6	5.4	2.43
1961	495.8	17,740.5	2.8	552.1	5.3	1.98
1962	579.5	19,314.8	3.0	649.6	9.8	3.50
1963	675.9	22,453.8	3.0	742.7	5.2	1.73
1964	845.0	25,636.4	3.3	919.5	7.8	2.54

Source: Japan, Ministry of Finance, Tax Bureau, *An Outline of Japanese Taxes*
(Tokyo: 1965); and National Planning Office of Japan.

The conclusion which follows from the above discussion is that in Japan,
as for the three continental European countries, the personal income tax
rather than being a stabilizer is a destabilizer. The reason for this perverse
reaction is, again, to be found in the method of assessment whereby the
incomes other than wages and salaries—which in 1963 accounted for 43.2 per
cent of the total tax—are subjected to the self-assessment system. This system
makes the tax payments in year t depend on the incomes in the year t-1.
Therefore, if year t-1 is a recession year but t is a boom year, the ratio of the
tax to the gross national product is bound to be low; the opposite will happen
when t-1 is a boom year and t a recession year.

UNITED KINGDOM

General Characteristics

Table VII-11 summarizes the historical relationship between the combined
revenues from the income tax and surtax on individuals and the gross national
product for the United Kingdom. The ratio of these revenues to the gross
national product shows a substantial increase going from 6.7 in 1953 to 9.2 in
1965. This increase is of particular significance coming in the face of a decrease of about 2 per cent in the total tax burden.

During the period considered, there were several changes in the rates or in
the size of the reliefs or allowances; the most important of these took place in
1955, 1956, 1959, and 1963. In 1955 and 1956 the standard rate was reduced from 45 to 42.5 per cent while, at the same time, many of the reliefs
and allowances were increased. In 1959 the standard rate was decreased once

TABLE VII-11. RELATIONSHIP BETWEEN PERSONAL INCOME TAXES
AND GNP FOR THE UNITED KINGDOM, 1953-65

(£ in millions)

Years	GNP[a] (1)	Income tax and surtax (2)	$\frac{T}{GNP}$ (3)	$\frac{\Delta T}{\Delta GNP}$ (4)	$\frac{\Delta T/T}{\Delta GNP/GNP}$ (5)
1953	17,005	1,134	6.7%	–	–
1954	17,948	1,236	6.9	10.8%	1.62%
1955	19,240	1,330	6.9	7.3	1.06
1956	20,893	1,452	6.9	7.4	1.07
1957	22,088	1,602	7.3	12.6	1.83
1958	23,054	1,696	7.4	9.7	1.33
1959	24,271	1,776	7.3	6.6	0.89
1960	25,699	2,001	7.8	15.8	2.16
1961	27,426	2,259	8.2	14.9	1.91
1962	28,738	2,469	8.6	16.0	1.95
1963	30,505	2,507	8.2	2.2	0.26
1964	32,994	2,750	8.3	9.8	1.20
1965	35,351	3,250	9.2	21.2	2.55

[a]Including taxes on expenditures levied on imports.

Source: Great Britain, Central Statistical Office, *National Income and Expenditure, 1966* (London: H.M.S.O.).

again to 38.75 per cent. In 1963 there were substantial increases in some of the allowances and reliefs.

Cyclical Behavior

The above reforms need to be kept in mind in looking at the estimates of the elasticities and flexibilities in Table VII-11. A comparison of column (4) with column (3) shows that for all but two years $\frac{\Delta T}{\Delta GNP} > \frac{T}{GNP}$. The two years for which this is not true—1959 and 1963— witnessed substantial reductions either in the rates or in the allowances. This implies that the British individual income tax has an elasticity greater than one.

For the United Kingdom there are two published studies on the sensitivity of the taxes on income to changes in national income. The first of these studies,[11] which relates the revenue from these taxes to personal incomes, concluded that "the stabilizing effect of the yield flexibility of personal income taxes [is] twenty per cent."[12] The second study[13] found that for 1957-58 the elasticity of the income tax yield with respect to income was

[11]P. H. Pearse, "Automatic Stabilization and the British Taxes on Income," *Review of Economic Studies*, February 1962, pp. 124-37.

[12]*Ibid.*, p. 137.

[13]A. R. Prest, "The Sensitivity of the Yield of Personal Income Tax in the United Kingdom," *The Economic Journal*, September 1962, pp. 576-96.

slightly over 2.1, and that the marginal income tax rate at 1959-60 rates was about .18 or about twice the average rate of tax for that year.[14]

The estimates by both Pearse and Prest are very close to those shown for the three years 1960-62 during which there was no important legislative change. Since the estimates in the table are related to the gross national product rather than to personal income, they are slightly lower.

In the United Kingdom also, the method of collection of the taxes probably reduces the built-in flexibility of the yield in a recession. In fact, while the P.A.Y.E. system is an almost perfect synchronism between earning of income and paying of taxes, the same is not true for the surtax for which there is a lag of about a year between earning of income and paying of the tax. Therefore, if a recession year follows a boom year, while the taxes out of the lower levels of wages and salaries would immediately decline, those on the other incomes would remain high; in fact, as a proportion of the incomes earned in the recession year, they would increase. This factor may have played a role in 1958 and 1962 which were recession years but during which, even though there was no legislative reform, the average tax rate reached very high levels.

UNITED STATES

A Method for Measuring the Income Sensitivity of the Individual Income Tax in the United States

Like the individual income tax of the other countries analyzed, that of the United States is essentially elastic. The ratio of the tax to the gross national product increased almost constantly from 7.3 per cent to 8.2 per cent between 1954 and 1963, although its nominal characteristics remained unchanged. During these nine years, the ratio fell during the years of recessions. There is no doubt that this tax provides a powerful stabilizer for the United States economy.

During the last few years, the sensitivity of this tax to changes in national income has been analyzed in several studies.[15] Although these studies have

---

[14]*Ibid.,* pp. 587 and 591.

[15]See inter alia: J. A. Pechman, "Yield of the Individual Income Tax during a Recession," N.B.E.R., *Policies to Combat Depression* (Princeton: Princeton University Press, 1956); L. J. Cohen, "An Empirical Measurement of the Built-in Flexibility of the Individual Income Tax," *American Economic Review,* May 1959; L. J. Cohen, "A more Recent Measurement of the Built-in Flexibility of the Individual Income Tax," *National Tax Journal,* June 1960; Richard Goode, *The Individual Income Tax* (Washington, D.C.: The Brookings Institution, 1964), Chapter XI and appendix E; Wilfred Lewis, Jr., *Federal Fiscal Policy in the Post-War Recessions* (Washington, D.C.: The Brookings Institution, 1962); James S. Duesenberry, Otto Eckstein, and Gary Fromm, "A Simulation of the United States Economy in Recession," *Econometrica,* Vol. 28, October 1960. For an earlier study, see R. A. Musgrave and M. H. Miller, "Built-in Flexibility," *American Economic Review,* Vol. 38, No. 1, March 1948.

differed in the details of their approach and in their degree of sophistication, basically they have attempted to measure that sensitivity by means of time-series approaches—by observing the reaction of the tax to actual or simulated changes in some aggregate estimate of national or personal income over a period of time. Such an approach, although sophisticated, has limitations that are unavoidable for estimates made at different points in time—for example, those owing to population changes. The a priori measure of the sensitivity of the personal income tax should be measured at a specific moment in time and if possible should be related to per capita estimates.[16]

In the following pages I suggest a method for estimating the sensitivity of the tax to changes in income—by using cross-section data at the state level. There are available annual data on per capita personal income, aggregate gross income, taxable income, and tax for the fifty states. The per capita personal income ranged, in 1963, from a high of $3,386 for Nevada to a low of $1,390 for Mississippi. Since each state was subjected to the same prevailing Federal income tax legislation, the substantial range of income covered by the states provides a way for analyzing the sensitivity of the United States' personal income tax over an equivalent range.

More specifically, assume that each state embodies all the economic and demographic characteristics of the United States and can, thus, be considered a random observation of the United States: a micro-United States. Then, for a given year, the relationship between the tax and the income for the fifty states may be considered as being equivalent to one obtained from fifty random observations, from time-series, for the United States for which the nominal tax system remains the same while the per capita income changes over the range given above. Of course, there will be some factors such as income distribution, industrial composition of income, demographic characteristics of each state's population and so on, which may make the observation on a particular state non-random. However, it is hoped that these factors, when they are not averaged out, are not important enough to bias the results.

Description of Data. The basic data[17] for the analysis are:

Y_p: per capita personal income
T: Federal income tax revenue

[16]Two studies which have relied on cross-section data using a different approach from the one used below are: E. J. Mishan and L. A. Dicks-Mireaux, "Progressive Taxation in an Inflationary Economy," *American Economic Review,* September 1958; and J. O. Blackburn, "Implicit Tax Rate Deductions with Growth, Progressive Taxes, Constant Progressivity, and a Fixed Public Share," *American Economic Review,* March 1967.

[17]The tax data were obtained from, U.S. Treasury Department, Internal Revenue Service, *Statistics of Income . . . 1963;* the data on personal income and population come from, U.S. Department of Commerce, *Statistical Abstract of the United States, 1965.*

TI: taxable income
AGI: adjusted gross income
P: population

Some aspects of the data confirm, through a completely different route, some conclusions reached by other investigators on the Federal income tax.

For example, consider Goode's conclusions in his analysis of the relationship between individual income tax and individual income for a period of several years. One aspect of that relationship that he found "somewhat peculiar"[18] is the constancy of the effective tax rate on taxable income at constant statutory rates. He concluded that from 1954 to 1960 "the average effective rate and average marginal rate (both computed with respect to taxable income) appear to have been approximately constant at about 23 per cent."[19]

The data confirmed Goode's findings to a surprising degree. Out of fifty states, only three (Nevada, Delaware, and New York) have a T/TI which is greater than 24 (and two of these three states were just over 24), and only seven have ratios lower than 22. Thus, forty out of fifty states have effective tax rates on taxable incomes between 22 and 24; 47 have a T/TI between 21 and 25. The states for which the T/TI ratio is smaller than 22 are not, generally, the poorest but, rather, the agricultural ones.

Unlike the relation between T and TI, which does not seem to be affected to any significant degree by the change in per capita personal income, that between TI and AGI is highly dependent on it. In fact, it increases almost continuously with income, going from about 47 per cent for Mississippi to above 61 per cent for some of the states with the highest per capita income.

Recalling that $\frac{T}{AGI} = \frac{T}{TI} \times \frac{TI}{AGI}$, it is immediately realized that, given the nominal structure, the average tax rate with respect to taxable income $\left(\frac{T}{TI}\right)$ plays almost no role in the determination of the changes in the average tax rate with respect to AGI (i.e., T/AGI); changes in T/AGI are almost totally dependent on changes in TI/AGI. This, again, confirms a conclusion already reached with time-series data.

Estimate of Flexibility and Elasticity. An application of regression analysis makes it possible to estimate the built-in flexibility and the elasticity of the Federal individual income tax in 1963. In its most common definition, the built-in flexibility with respect to AGI is given by the expression:[20]

[18]Goode, R. *op. cit.,* p. 291.

[19]*Ibid.*

[20]This is the definition used by Pechman and Cohen in the works listed on p. 105, footnote 15.

$$\frac{\Delta T}{\Delta AGI} = \frac{\Delta TI}{\Delta AGI} \times \frac{\Delta T}{\Delta TI} \cdot$$

$\frac{\Delta TI}{\Delta AGI}$ can be estimated from an equation of the type $\frac{TI}{P} = a + b\frac{AGI}{P}$, and

$\frac{\Delta T}{\Delta TI}$ from an equation of the type $\frac{T}{P} = a + b\frac{TI}{P}$. The estimated regression lines are:

(1) $\frac{TI}{P} = -270.7302 + 0.7070\frac{AGI}{P}$

(0.0087)

$r^2 = 0.9886$

(2) $\frac{T}{P} = -23.1109 + 0.2508\frac{TI}{P}$

(0.0055)

$r^2 = 0.9777$

The estimate of the built-in flexibility, then, is

$$\frac{\Delta T}{\Delta AGI} = (0.7070)(0.2508) = 0.1775.$$

An alternative way of estimating the built-in flexibility from the data in the table is by regressing directly the tax against AGI; i.e., by using an equation of the type $\frac{T}{P} = a + b\frac{AGI}{P}$. The estimated regression line is then,

(3) $\frac{T}{P} = -89.2039 + 0.1763\frac{AGI}{P}$

(0.0046)

$r^2 = 0.9557$

which gives practically the same estimate for the flexibility.

In the estimated equations obtained above, the form of the relationship has been assumed to be linear. A priori, however, in view of the progressivity of the income tax, one would expect that relationship to be nonlinear. In view of this, the exponential form $T = AY^\beta$ is preferable. In this form, the function appears as a straight line with $\log A$ as the vertical intercept and β as the slope of the straight line which is also the elasticity of T with respect to Y. The equation thus obtained is:

$$\log\frac{T}{P} = -2.14328 + 1.38138\log\frac{AGI}{P}$$

(0.04401)

$r^2 = 0.95453$

It can be seen that the elasticity of this tax with respect to adjusted gross income is about 1.38 which means that a 1 per cent increase or decrease in AGI results in a 1.38 per cent increase or decrease in the tax revenues. Knowing the elasticity, and the ratio of the tax revenue to adjusted gross income for 1963, the flexibility of the tax, which is the product of the two,[21] can be easily determined. Thus $\frac{\Delta T}{\Delta AGI} = E_T \times \frac{T}{AGI} = (1.38138)$ (13.07) = 18.037, which is very close to the estimates obtained above.

In 1963, AGI was 62.6 per cent of the gross national product which implies that if the flexibility were related to the gross national product it would be about 11.1 per cent. The estimates obtained here are slightly higher than those obtained by most of the other studies.[22] However, all of those other estimates are for earlier years; given a certain rate structure, the flexibility of the individual income tax can be expected to increase with the passing of time.

CONCLUSION

The analysis of the relationship between the personal income tax and the gross national product of the countries has shown that Japan, with the fastest rate of growth, is also the only one where the percentage of the tax to the gross national product has decreased: from 4.1 in 1953 to 3.3 in 1964. On the other hand the United Kingdom, with the slowest rate of growth, is the one in which that percentage has increased the most: from 6.7 in 1953 to 9.2 in 1965. For Germany, the percentage remained almost constant during the period of highest growth; it went from 5.95 in 1953 to 6.03 in 1960, but increased rather steeply in the last few years when the growth rate has been slower: from 1960 to 1964 it increased from 6.03 to 7.58, and decreased again—to 7.33—in 1965. In Italy, France, and the United States, the increase has been only about 1 percentage point for the last decade.

These results raise the obvious question whether or not there was any relation between the growth performance of these economies and the behavior of the actual income tax burdens. In this connection, it is important to point out that in the absence of any governmental action, the countries which increased fastest are those which should have shown the largest increase in the T/GNP ratio. The fact that they did not was the result of fiscal policies aimed at reducing the revenues from this tax; in other words, it was the result of frequent tax cuts. That such tax cuts do stimulate the aggregate

---

[21]Since the elasticity is $E_T = \left(\frac{\Delta T}{T}\right)\left(\frac{\Delta AGI}{AGI}\right) = \left(\frac{\Delta T}{\Delta AGI}\right)\left(\frac{AGI}{T}\right)$ and the flexibility is $\frac{\Delta T}{\Delta AGI}$, the latter can be obtained by multiplying E_T by $\frac{T}{AGI}$; or $\frac{\Delta T}{\Delta AGI} = \left(\frac{\Delta T}{\Delta AGI}\right)\left(\frac{AGI}{T}\right)\left(\frac{T}{AGI}\right)$.

[22]For example, Cohen's estimate for 1954-57 was 14.5 with respect to AGI and 8.2 with respect to GNP. Pechman's estimate was 17.55 at 1953 tax rates and between 15 per cent and 16 per cent at 1954 rates; in relation to GNP, the latter percentages would be between 8.4 and 9.0. Goode's estimate with respect to GNP is 8.7.

demand and help to move the economy close to a full-employment rate of growth is theoretically obvious and has been convincingly demonstrated by the American experiment of 1964.[23] One can safely conclude that the tax-cut policy of Japan or the frequent tax reforms of Germany (up to 1958) and France did remove an obstacle from the path of growth and thus permitted that growth to take place. One should not, however, claim more than this. One cannot realistically attribute the Japanese growth to the tax-cut policy, although without that policy such a growth might not have been possible. Equally, one cannot attribute the low growth rate of the United Kingdom to the increase in the income tax burden, although the economy would have been better off without that increase or with a decrease.

Apart from the behavior of the *T/GNP* ratio over the period considered, there are other aspects of the income taxes which should be considered here in relation to the growth of the countries.. Built-in flexibility, while it may be a "blessing" during a recession, can become an obstacle to growth due to the tendency of revenues from the personal income tax to increase faster than the gross national product. One can point to the fact that the country with the highest flexibility—the United Kingdom—was the one with the slowest rate of growth. Given a certain elasticity, the more important the income tax in a country is, the greater will be its flexibility and the greater the dampening effect on growth even when the economy is growing from a less than full-employment level. Therefore, in growing countries it is particularly important that frequent tax cuts take place.

In connection with the alleged stabilizing effects of the income tax over the cycle, the conclusion which follows from this chapter is that, since most of the writing on the built-in flexibility of the income tax has been done in the United States, the importance of the method of collection, especially with regard to synchronousness, has not been sufficiently emphasized. Only in the United States did such a synchronism take place. All the other countries, to different degrees, showed collections which lagged behind the earning of the income. For this reason the effectiveness of the tax to dampen a downswing, or for that matter an upswing, is lower than one would expect from the importance of the tax and in some of the countries the tax could very will be considered a destabilizer.

---

[23]For a discussion of this point see, for example, David J. Ott and Attiat F. Ott, *Federal Budget Policy* (Washington, D.C.: The Brookings Institution, 1964).

VIII

INDIVIDUAL INCOME TAXATION AND
PERSONAL SAVINGS

Personal income taxation is considered to have a negative influence on growth through its effect on saving. Generally, all taxes, by decreasing the disposable income of the taxpayer, can be expected to decrease saving. Disposable income, however, can be saved or consumed; while almost any tax is paid partly out of consumption and partly out of saving, it is often argued that a tax on personal income decreases personal saving more than one on consumption. If this assumption is correct, then it is justifiable to believe that personal saving in the countries which have relied heavily on personal income taxation should have been more affected than in the other countries.

There are, however, many factors which influence and determine the propensity to save on the part of the household sector, and taxation is just one of them. It would indeed be surprising if it were so important that one could find statistically significant relationships, except in very unusual circumstances, between personal saving and personal income taxes. An analysis of this relationship must aim at showing the aspects of the personal income taxes which may be expected to be important.

There are three aspects which, apart from the weight of the tax, ought to be considered. First and most obvious are the specific measures introduced by some of the countries which attempt to increase particular forms of savings in the hope that this will increase total personal saving rather than just change its composition. Second, there are the effects on personal saving which arise out of differential tax treatment of different kinds of income. Third, there is the progressivity of the tax which is also relevant to the propensity to save.

TAX MEASURES TO STIMULATE PERSONAL SAVINGS

The increase of personal savings has been one of the explicit objectives of tax policy in three of the countries considered: France, Germany, and Japan. There has been a belief among the tax authorities of these countries that, by providing some special tax treatment on some specific forms of uses of income, personal saving could be made to increase. It may be worthwhile to look into the most important of these measures to see if, and/or to what extent, they can provide an explanation for the difference in the propensity of the personal sector to save.

France

Since 1950 French tax policy has accepted the principle that personal saving should not be taxed. This principle has had a long list of outstanding defenders and there can be no doubt that Nicholas Kaldor was right in writing that "there can be few ideas in the field of economics which are so revolutionary in their implication, and yet can look back on so respectable an ancestry."[1] Its acceptance on the part of the French tax authority has not been accompanied by its incorporation in the tax system, but some attempts have been made in that direction. The value-added tax is defended along these lines.

In the specific area of personal income taxation, the acceptance of the principle has, so far, manifested itself in the introduction of various exemptions from the individual income tax. These include the interest on Treasury bills and other government securities, interest on deposits in the national savings bank system (*Caisse d'Epargne*), interest on bonds issued by the national agricultural bank, the deduction allowed to life insurance premiums (on condition that the policy was taken before January 1, 1959). This last deduction is usually subjected to the limit of 10 per cent of the declared net income with a limit of F400 increased by F100 per dependent. Whenever the insurance contract was for at least ten years, the deductions allowed are F2,000 plus F400 per dependent. Other important deductions are those connected with the payment of interest on construction loans for the first ten years. The limit for this latter deduction is F5,000 for each dependent. On September 16, 1964 the government announced that, in order to stimulate saving, the first F500 of income from bonds and debentures would also not be taxed. This measure is to remain in effect from January 1, 1965 to December 31, 1970.

The general belief with respect to these measures is that although the French authorities have attempted to influence the flow of personal saving, the income involved has been so small that the effect that these tax measures may have had on personal saving may be assumed to have been marginal.

Germany

In Germany, on the other hand, the tax measures to stimulate total saving have been very important and the effect of these measures on investment

---

[1]Nicholas Kaldor, *An Expenditure Tax* (London: George Allen & Unwin Ltd, 1955), p. 12.

quite considerable. As far as *personal* saving is concerned, its reaction to tax incentive probably became important only after 1955; up to that year, the intensity of the war—induced demand together with the congenital fear of inflation did not leave much scope for personal saving especially in liquid form. Up to 1958 the main objective of these measures was to increase saving to make it equal to *ex-ante* investment at the current rates of interest. Since 1958, the objective has been more and more that of redistributing wealth.

The types of savings which the German tax incentives have tried to promote can be classified[2] as (a) savings with insurance, (b) savings earmarked for construction of dwellings, (c) direct savings accounts, (d) saving by acquisition of securities. By and large, all these types of savings have been deductible from taxable income with some limitations. The amounts which may be deducted are shown in Table VIII-1. In 1959, tax exemptions for savings accounts and for securities were abolished and replaced by government premiums to private savers. The premium is equivalent to 20 per cent of savings not withdrawn for five years and is limited to only DM600 per year for a single person and DM1,200 for married couples. For persons over fifty years of age the premiums are doubled.

TABLE VIII-1. YEARLY SAVINGS DEDUCTIBLE FROM TAXABLE INCOME
IN GERMANY (in DM)

Regulations for persons under 50 years of age	Single person	Married couple	Each child
1959 to Date:			
Initial maximum deductible	1,100	2,200	500
Maximum of increment half deductible	1,100	2,200	500
Total amount deductible	1,650	3,300	750
1949-54, initial maximum deductible	800	1,200	400
1955, initial maximum deductible	800	1,600	500
1956-58, initial maximum deductible	1,000	2,000	500

Source: Karl Häuser, "West Germany," N.B.E.R. and The Brookings Institution, *Foreign Tax Policies and Economic Growth* (New York: Columbia University Press, 1966), p. 126.

The amounts which are subjected to these tax privileges were quite sizable[3] as were the costs of those tax incentives to the government which in 1962 reached DM1,427 million.

The obvious question that has been asked is whether these incentives have succeeded in increasing total personal saving apart from the impact that they

[2]See Karl Häuser, "West Germany," N.B.E.R. and The Brookings Institution, *Foreign Tax Policies and Economic Growth* (New York: Columbia University Press, 1966), p. 126.
[3]*Ibid.*, p. 127.

may have had on its composition. According to Häuser, their impact on personal saving has been marginal while they have cost the government a considerable amount of money.

Japan

In Japan the need for additional savings to meet the growing investment demand has been manifested by the "reinforcement of personal saving policy," according to which many types of property income have been favored. Thus, the increase of personal saving has been an explicit objective of the Japanese tax policy. The most important among the provisions adopted to achieve this objective are the following:[4]

1. *Tax exemption of interest income from small deposits.* According to this provision, whenever the principal of a saving deposit does not exceed a specified limit (500,000 yen in 1963), the interest is exempted from the personal income tax.[5] Up to 1963, when for the first time the saving institutions were required to report the names of the depositors, anyone could evade the tax by depositing his savings in several banks in such a way that no deposit exceeded the prescribed maximum.

2. *Separate low taxation of interest income.* Between 1955 and 1957 interest income was completely exempted from the tax. Since 1957 it has been taxed at very low rates (10 per cent up to 1963 and 5 per cent since then). This incentive has been particularly beneficial to the higher income groups since, as it has been seen above, the interest income from small saving deposits were already exempted. The fraction of total savings which benefited from this low rate was 21.7 per cent in 1960.

3. *Favorable treatment of dividend income.* As with interest income, income from dividends also benefits from special treatments. There has been, over the last decade, a substantial reduction in the tax rate which applies to some forms of dividend income ("distribution of gains of a securities investment trust") from 20 per cent until 1955, to 10 per cent, and then, again, in 1963 to 5 per cent. The tax on these dividends is withheld at the source. Furthermore, 15 per cent of dividend income other than the one above may be deducted from the taxpayer's total income (7.5 per cent if the total income exceeds 10 million yen).[6] This measure is particularly advantageous to high income classes since the fifth quintile in the income distribution is reported to own over 70 per cent of the total value of stocks[7] but less than 50 per cent of the total saving deposits.

[4] See Ryutaro Komiya, "Japan," *Foreign Tax Policies, op. cit.,* pp. 56-63.

[5] For details see Japan, Ministry of Finance, Tax Bureau, *An Outline of Japanese Taxes* (Tokyo: 1964), pp. 38-39.

[6] *Ibid.,* pp. 43-46.

[7] Japan, Bureau of Statistics, Prime Minister's Office, *Survey of Trends in Saving for 1960 and 1961* (Tokyo), pp. 127-28.

4. *Deduction of life insurance premiums.* Life insurance premiums are also exempted from the personal income tax subject to a limit which, from 2,000 yen in 1951, has increased to 15,000 yen plus half of the excess over 15,000 yen up to 35,000 yen.

The above described privileged treatment of some incomes has caused a substantial erosion of the personal income tax base for incomes other than those from wages and salaries, with inevitable losses to tax revenues and consequent inequities. These losses in the periods between 1958 and 1963 have averaged about 15 per cent of the total personal income tax revenues.

In view of the considerable scope of these privileges, one must ask if they did have an effect on the volume (again as distinguished from the composition) of personal saving. Komiya distinguishes three possible effects: the interest elasticity of saving, the income redistribution effect, and the evasion effect.

With respect to the first, he writes that "the basic theory implicit in these special tax provisions is that the elasticity of the supply of personal saving is substantially greater than zero. The theory is dubious on theoretical and empirical ground."[8] He maintains that "the average Japanese saver does not seem to be sensitive to small changes in the interest rate."[9] In view of this, he concludes that the effect on savings may have been zero.

One can argue with him, however, on the ground that the revenue losses due to the exemption of savings from taxation probably were compensated by increases in other taxes; either taxes on nonexempted income or indirect taxes must have been made higher than they would have been if the privileges had not been enacted. Thus, the *after-tax* ratio of property income to the total income of the average taxpayer increased; the effect is the same as if no privileges had been granted but the size of the property of the average taxpayer had increased. If it is assumed that this kind of increase in wealth did not affect consumption, then the net effect was probably an increase in saving. Komiya is aware of this effect, but he connects it exclusively with a redistribution of income. He writes in fact that:

To the extent that higher income families receive a higher proportion of their income from property holding, favorable treatment of property income makes income distribution more unequal. If it is assumed that the marginal propensity to save is higher for higher income families, favorable tax treatment of property income has a positive effect on the total supply of personal saving.[10]

[8]Komiya, *op. cit.*, p. 60.
[9]*Ibid.*
[10]*Ibid.*, p. 62.

Finally, he mentions that there may have been a tax evasion effect if the taxpayers who could evade the tax more easily also had a higher marginal propensity to save. His conclusion is that, if personal saving increased, it was because of the adverse redistributive effects which the privileges caused.

PROGRESSIVITY OF THE PERSONAL INCOME TAX AND PERSONAL SAVING

In some of the discussions about the relative effects on growth of direct and indirect taxes, it has been maintained that personal saving in the United States and the United Kingdom has been reduced by their greater reliance on personal income taxes and that this reduction has been a factor in their slower growth rates.

There are theoretical arguments and empirical studies which indicate that the impact of a given level of taxation on personal saving depends on the type of tax that is imposed; however, those arguments indicate that the issue of personal saving is related to the choice between progressive and non-progressive taxes rather than between personal income and sales taxes. Therefore, the personal income tax burdens, per se, do not tell anything about the relative saving-reducing effects of the tax systems of these countries. To illustrate this point I will rely on some empirical findings for the United States.

Some studies have indicated that in the United States the Federal individual income tax reduces personal saving more than does a proportional income tax of the same yield; the latter, in turn, reduces personal saving more than an equivalent flat-rate general sales tax. Thus, according to two studies, the proportions of tax revenues which can be assumed to be paid out of personal savings are as shown below:

	Musgrave[11] (1957)	Goode[12] (1950)
Federal individual income tax	31	33
Proportional income tax	22	28
Sales tax	18	27

These differential effects on personal savings are basically a reflection of differences in marginal propensity to save among the various income groups.

[11] Richard Musgrave, "Effects of Tax Policy on Private Capital Formation," *Fiscal and Debt Management Policies,* Research Studies for the Commission on Money and Credit (Englewood Cliffs, N.J.: Prentice-Hall, 1963), pp. 65-68.

[12] Richard Goode, *The Individual Income Tax* (Washington, D.C.: The Brookings Institution, 1964), p. 67.

In other words, they are the consequence of the increase of the marginal propensity to save with respect to income.

If Musgrave's estimates are considered more realistic—since they refer to a more recent year—and, if those estimates, based on the year 1957, were still valid in 1963, then the United States personal saving would have been, in 1963, $6.27 billion, or 30.7 per cent, higher if the revenues from the progressive income tax had been levied with a sales tax; and $4.34 billion, or 21.2 per cent, higher if the same revenues had been collected by means of a proportional income tax.

As these estimates show, about two-thirds of the losses in saving are *not* a consequence of the use of personal income taxes instead of sales taxes but, specifically, of *progressive* personal income taxes. Therefore, it is not sufficient to argue that the greater use of income taxes reduced their savings by a larger proportion. The argument must instead be based on the greater "progressivity" of these taxes vis-a-vis other taxes, since the higher income taxes in the United States and the United Kingdom were not a net addition to total tax revenues, rather, they could be assumed to have replaced other taxes, and most likely taxes of an indirect nature. If the American and British income tax revenues had been collected with proportional income taxes, most of the argument would fall apart.

Furthermore, in Musgrave's estimates, the saving-reducing effect of the progressive income tax is compared with that of a flat-rate sales tax. However, most of the sales and excise taxes which can be assumed to have taken the place of the individual income tax in the countries which rely least on the latter are not flat-rate general sales taxes but, in general, taxes on luxuries more than on necessities. Therefore, ceteris paribus, the gains in savings to these countries are probably lower than what one would expect from Musgrave's estimates.

I shall proceed with a kind of simulation exercise by applying Musgrave's estimates to the income tax revenues of some of the other countries to get an idea of how the personal savings of these countries may have been affected. This is, of course, just an exercise but it probably gives realistic estimates as to the magnitudes that can be expected. I will draw on the results of Chapter IV for estimates of the progressivity of the income taxes.

The Italian system is undoubtedly the most favorable to personal saving since only about 15 per cent of the national income is taxed with a progressive tax at an average rate of only about 3 per cent. The revenue from this tax was only .5 per cent of the national income. Therefore, even if all of this revenue had been paid out of personal saving, the latter would have been reduced by a rather insignificant proportion. Unfortunately, neither personal saving nor personal income data are available for Italy, so that the contribution of the households to total saving is not known. However, in view of the smallness of the corporate sector and of the national gross saving rate of about 25 per cent, personal saving must have been substantial.

At the other extreme of the spectrum one must inevitably put the United Kingdom. In this country, the ratio of the personal income tax to the personal income is about 10 per cent. Furthermore, this is by far the most progressive of all the income taxes analyzed in this study. For example, the top 3.6 per cent of the taxpayers (with incomes over £2,000 and receiving about 16.2 per cent of the taxable income) in 1963, paid 44.4 per cent of the total tax. In the United States, on the other hand, the top 4.8 per cent of the taxpayers paid only about 25 per cent of the tax. According to one study[13] for an earlier year, the top decile of the before-tax income saved 23.5 per cent in the United States compared with 9.9 per cent in the United Kingdom. While these results could be attributed to many factors, it would seem that the progressivity of the income tax plays an important role.

Conservatively, I will assume that more than 40 per cent of the income tax revenues are paid out of potential savings in the United Kingdom. Using this estimate it can be calculated that if the same revenues had been levied with a flat-rate sales tax, and if the saving-reducing effect of the sales tax were the same as for the United States, personal saving, in 1964, would have been about £576 million higher, or about one-third of *gross* personal saving.

For the other countries, the evidence is less clear-cut. Figure IV-1 on page 39 shows that the Japanese tax is quite progressive, with 2 per cent of the taxpayers paying 33.5 per cent of the tax. However, the revenue from this tax is relatively small (574 billion yen in 1963). Therefore, even if the share paid out of saving were as great as that of the British tax (that is, if it is assumed that 40 per cent of it was paid out of potential savings), a shift from this tax to an equal-yield, flat-rate sales tax would increase personal saving by only 126.3 billion yen or by about 4.2 per cent assuming that, as in the United States, 18 per cent of the yield of the sales tax would have been paid out of saving. Furthermore if, for the sake of discussion, it is assumed that the ratio of the revenue from the income tax were in Japan the same proportion of personal income as in the United States (this would imply increasing it from 574 billion yen to 1,435 billion yen in 1963), and if the progressivity of the income tax in Japan were the same as for the United States, then a shift to a flat-rate, sales tax—given Musgrave's estimates—would increase savings by 186.6 billion yen or by only 6.2 per cent.

In France, the revenue from the progressive income tax in 1963 was about F12 billion collected with effective rates at least as progressive as those for the American income tax. To get the same ratio of the tax to the personal income as in the United States, France should have collected about F35

[13]J. B. Lansing and H. Lydall, "An Anglo-American Comparison of Personal Saving," *Bulletin of the Oxford Institute of Statistics,* August 1960.

billion. In view of the over all high tax burden for France, one can assume that the difference between F35 billion and F12 billion—or F23 billion—was collected as sales taxes. Now the question to ask is: By how much would French personal saving have been lower had that F23 billion been collected through a progressive income tax? If Musgrave's estimates are also applied here the answer would be about F3 billion—or 13 per cent of F23 billion. Thus, personal saving would have been about 12.8 per cent lower than it was.

For Germany, the ratio of the revenue from the income tax to personal income was somewhat lower than in the United States and the United Kingdom for most of the postwar period. Furthermore, the various reforms greatly reduced the progressivity of this tax. Thus, up to about 1958, the reduction in potential savings due to the payment of the income tax was probably just about what it would have been if a sales tax had been in use instead. However, the situation changed after 1958. In more recent years, although the nominal rates for the high income brackets were still somewhat lower than in the United States, the effective average rates for most of the income brackets were probably as high. Thus, the share of the personal income tax paid out of saving must have been increasing and now it may very well be as high as in the United States.

The point of the above exercise is that while heavy reliance on the progressive income taxes does normally involve a decrease in personal saving, it is very easy to exaggerate that decrease. It must be realized that, apart from Japan and the United States, the countries which are being compared have approximately equivalent total tax burdens. Therefore, the lower revenues from income taxes in countries such as Italy, France, and, to a lesser extent, Germany were compensated by higher indirect taxes. Indirect taxes also reduce saving although normally less than progressive income taxes. Furthermore, the revenues from the income taxes, except for Italy, were normally collected with effective rates which were as progressive as in the United States.

From the analysis of this section, it may be concluded that the different reliance on income taxes did play a role in the determination of the personal sector's propensity to save, but it was not an overwhelming one. For example, it would be absurd to argue that in Japan, increasing the ratio of the income tax to personal income, while decreasing the other taxes by an equivalent amount (from about 4 per cent to the level of the United States and the United Kingdom—i.e., about 10 per cent), could have reduced the average propensity to save of the personal sector from over 20 per cent to anywhere near the American or British level of about 7 per cent.

However, while the importance of this factor should not be exaggerated, it should not be minimized either. In the United Kingdom, the combination of the importance and the progressivity of the tax did reduce saving by a significant level. The United States tax, on the other hand, turns out to be, in effect, not more progressive than the taxes of the other countries except Italy. Since, apart from Japan, those countries had total tax burdens somewhat heavier than the United States, it is conceivable to assume that the other taxes compensated for the lighter income tax burden. Thus, in conclusion, with the possible exception of Italy and Japan, it is possible that personal saving was not reduced more in the United States than in the other countries.

INCOME TAX TREATMENT OF DIFFERENT KINDS OF INCOME AND PERSONAL SAVING

The third aspect of the relation between income taxation and personal saving which ought to be considered is the tax treatment of different kinds of incomes. This aspect was discussed at length in a previous chapter; therefore, only a few remarks will be necessary here.

There is evidence to indicate that people with incomes from property and enterprise have a greater propensity to save than those with *equivalent* incomes from employment. Several reasons have been given for this difference in behavior. Houthakker[14] has suggested that the greater facility for reinvestment, which these incomes have, encourages saving. Friedman finds the main reason in the fact that the rate of return on saving from income from property and enterprise is normally much higher than for saving from labor income since the latter cannot, generally, be reinvested directly but must go through the capital market.[15] The uncertainty connected with non-contractual incomes (incomes from enterprises) is the reason given by Kaldor for those incomes to be saved more readily than contractual incomes (salaries).[16] Another reason may simply be that people whose wealth or property is not inherited may have accumulated it just because they had a low marginal propensity to consume; in other words the possession of property may itself be a function of a higher marginal propensity to save rather than the other way around.

Whichever the reason, it follows that, if property income is taxed more heavily than labor income, saving will suffer. It should be pointed out, however, that the empirical analysis of Chapter V does not really show how *equal* incomes from different sources are taxed. In fact, in the empirical conclusions of that chapter, both *type* of income and *level* of income played a role. Since property incomes are normally associated with higher levels of incomes, and

[14]H. S. Houthakker, "An International Comparison of Personal Savings," *International Statistical Bulletin,* May-June 1960.

[15]Milton Friedman, *Theory of the Consumption Function* (Princeton: Princeton University Press, 1957), p. 243.

[16]Nicholas Kaldor, "Alternative Theories of Distribution," *Review of Economic Studies,* No. 61, 1955-56.

since the income taxes are normally progressive, even in the absence of any discrimination against those incomes, they would still end up paying a higher average tax per dollar of income than the other incomes.

Keeping in mind the limitations of the results of Chapter V, the conclusions of that chapter as related to the present one can be reviewed briefly. For Japan, because of the difference in erosion which was due in part to the various schemes which allowed the exemption of much property and enterprise income, the average tax rate on incomes other than those from dependent labor was very low averaging, in 1963, only about 1.5 per cent. For France, too, the substantially greater erosion of incomes other than wages and salaries compensated to a large extent for the legal discrimination provided to wages and salaries so that the effective average tax rates on them were very low. In Italy, the situation was basically the same although here the effective tax rate on incomes other than wages and salaries, which was only 4.7 per cent, was somewhat higher than the 1.6 per cent on wages and salaries.

In the United Kingdom the effective rate on wages and salaries, approximately 8 per cent, was only about one-third of that on the other incomes, which were taxed with a rate several times as high as that for the same incomes in France, Italy, and Japan. In Germany, if 1963 is taken as the reference year, the situation approached that of the United Kingdom, although it was less extreme: the average rate for wages and salaries was a little higher than in the U.K., but somewhat lower for the other incomes. If an earlier year had been considered, the average rates on the two types of incomes would have been lower and not so different. Finally, for the United States this type of information is not available although, due to the apparently greater erosion for incomes other than wages and salaries, and due to the lack of legal discrimination in favor of the latter incomes, it is very unlikely that one would find differences in the average effective rates as high as in the United Kingdom.

CONCLUSION

Personal saving, though perhaps not as important as corporate saving for industrial growth, contributes substantially to the financing of new and fast-growing enterprises through its contribution to the capital market. If an economy is functioning at a full employment level, a reduction of personal saving may reduce the potential rate of growth. To the extent that this situation prevails, the impact of the income tax on personal saving becomes a factor to be taken into consideration in making policy decisions.

The evidence reviewed in this chapter indicates that Japan and Italy were probably the two countries where the personal income tax had the least negative impact on personal saving. Japan has gone further than any other country with its "reinforcement of personal saving policy" in providing means by which people with incomes other than wages and salaries could escape taxation; the outcome was that they paid almost no tax at all on those incomes. This general policy probably played a role in making Japanese households save over 20 per cent of their income. In Italy the three factors considered in this chapter were such to expect that the income tax would have a very low effect on personal saving: In the first place, the tax on individuals was very low: secondly, there was almost no progressivity in the effective rates and, thirdly, the rates on the types of incomes from which most of the saving may be expected to be generated were very low. However, no data are available on either personal saving or personal income in Italy.

In France the share of personal saving in relation to personal income has increased from about 2 per cent in the early 1950's to around 8 per cent after 1960. The French personal income tax was such that it must not have put any obstacle to such an increase since (a) the revenues from the tax were relatively low; (b) the effective rates on incomes other than wages and salaries were also very low; and (c) some measures were enacted to stimulate personal savings.

The United Kingdom is the country for which personal saving ought to have been reduced most by the personal income taxes. Here the progressivity of the tax was higher than in any other country and much of the revenue was collected with very high rates. Furthermore, the rates were particularly heavy on incomes other than wages and salaries and no provisions were available for the encouragement of savings.

For Germany it is important to make a distinction between the more recent years and the period of fastest growth of the economy. During the latter period several provisions for encouraging saving were available. Furthermore, the burden of the income tax was not too heavy, its rates were moderate and the difference between the average rates on wages and salaries and other incomes was relatively small. During this period the ratio of household saving to disposable income was high and growing, reaching a level of over 14 per cent for the period 1957-60. After 1960, however, that ratio not only stopped increasing, but it actually decreased. This change came at the same period when the effective rate of the tax on incomes other than wages and salaries increased substantially, giving support to the possibility that the developments in the income tax were having important negative effects on saving.

In the United States, the individual income taxes did reduce personal saving. That reduction was probably not as high as for the United Kingdom since the effective rates on most income brackets were not too high.

IX

INDIVIDUAL INCOME TAXATION AND
ECONOMIC GROWTH

It is now possible to draw some tentative conclusions about the relationship between the individual income tax and economic growth in the six countries studied. One would expect this relationship to be negative—that is, the growth rates will be lower for the countries that depend the most on the individual income tax as a source of revenue. But this expectation would be justified only if one could assume that, in the absence of the tax factor, the countries' capacity for growth would be exactly identical. This is, of course, an absurd assumption, as Denison's recent work[1] has clearly indicated. Quite apart from taxation, the factors which determine the rate of growth of the countries are not of the same intensity: Labor force, work hours, education, capital, technology, and so forth are normally changing at different rates, and thus the countries' capacity for growth are definitely not the same.

Taxation, then, must be considered as a significant element in the growth process to the extent that it makes the actual rates of growth diverge from the potential. The existence of income taxes will normally interfere with the growth process of the countries and will cause a decline in their growth rates. The extent of the decline will depend, of course, not only on the size of the tax but also on several of its structural characteristics. However, since one cannot know what the rates of growth of the various countries would have been in the absence of the income taxes, one cannot estimate that decline. But one can consider the various elements in the income tax of each country and relate them to the economic growth of the country. If it is found that the countries that experienced low rates of growth were also those in which the negative elements of the individual income taxes were predominant, while in the countries that grew faster those elements were either missing or not strong, then a dependence between taxation and growth would be assumed.

[1]Edward F. Denison (assisted by Jean-Pierre Poullier), *Why Growth Rates Differ* (Washington, D.C.: The Brookings Institution, 1967).

Table IX-1 indicates that the growth performance of the six countries was very uneven, with Japan growing at exceptional rates and the United Kingdom lagging far behind. The European countries did fairly well while the United States' performance was less satisfactory.

TABLE IX-1. ECONOMIC GROWTH IN THE SIX COUNTRIES, 1950-60
AND 1956-64

(percentages)

Countries	1950-60	1956-64
France	4.7	5.1
Germany	7.6	5.5
Italy	5.9	5.7
Japan	—	10.5
United Kingdom	2.6	3.3
United States	3.2	3.4

Source: O.E.C.D., *National Accounts Statistics* (Paris: O.E.C.D., annual).

The growth rates shown in the table are consistent with the findings of this study. The experiences of the United Kingdom and of Japan are perhaps the most significant. In the British case, it is evident that this tax had all the characteristics that would make it an obstacle to growth.

The burden of this tax was higher in the United Kingdom than in any other country; relative to income, more revenues were collected in this country than in any other. Unlike the United States and Germany, the method of collection was certainly detrimental to growth. Thus, the reason for arguing that the United Kingdom was affected most by the individual income tax depends not only on the size of that tax but also on its structure.

The British tax was characterized by high exemptions and allowances and by very high nominal and effective rates, so that most of the revenues were collected from the higher income classes with high marginal rates while the lower income classes paid very little. Apart from possible disincentive effects that such high rates may have had on the taxpayers' attitude toward work and investment, these rates affected personal savings, which play a fundamental role in the financing of new, growing enterprises unable to borrow in the capital market. Thus, the fact that in the aggregate there seems to have been no scarcity of saving for the established enterprises in no way changes the conclusion that the small and the new ones were negatively affected.

In addition, the spread between the average tax rate on incomes from wages and salaries and other types of income was far higher in the United Kingdom than in any other country. This was, to a certain extent, the result of high rates on high incomes, but it was also in part the result of legal discrimination against investment income. Such a discrimination may be justified on social, but certainly not on economic, grounds since it is bound to reduce personal saving.

The British individual income tax had one additional characteristic that would make it an obstacle to growth: its very high built-in flexibility. This is, of course, a desirable aspect in connection with mild fluctuations; however, it becomes "an ambiguous blessing"[2] when an economy suffers from a low growth rate.[3] In such cases the protection that it gives "against upward movements becomes an obstacle on the path to full employment, throttling expansion long before full employment is reached."[4] In the case of the British economy, which certainly did not show any exuberant character, the built-in flexibility was not an asset.

Japan, on the other hand, had an experience completely different from that of the United Kingdom. The Japanese tax, although it was far less burdensome than the British, showed a decrease in relation to gross national product over the period. Furthermore, it was collected mostly from wages and salaries; the average rates on other incomes were lower than on wages and salaries; and it did not have marginal rates as high as the British. Japan succeeded in greatly reducing the degree of erosion in spite of the decrease in the tax burden over the period, thus lowering the average tax rate on reported incomes. It also provided substantial incentives for personal saving.

For Germany, too, there was a relation between the economic performance and the personal income tax structure over the period. During the period of fastest growth (which ended around 1960), the burden of the individual income tax was not high and was either stable or decreasing: the divergence between the average tax rate on wages and salaries and on the other incomes was rather small; the exemptions were not too high and the progressivity quite limited with relatively low marginal rates; the tax reforms which took place kept the actual flexibility within limits; and many measures were instituted to stimulate personal saving and investment. After 1958, however, owing to the absence of important reforms, the ratio of the yield of the tax (or taxes) to the gross national product started to increase; the divergence between the average tax rate on wages and salaries and that on the other incomes became substantial with possible detrimental effects on personal savings; in view of the increase in per capita income, a larger share of the reported income came within the range of the progressivity of the rates; and the built-in flexibility acquired important values. Because of these changes

[2]U.S., Council of Economic Advisers, *Economic Report of the President,* (Washington, D.C.: G.P.O., 1963), p. 68.

[3]Richard Goode, *The Individual Income Tax* (Washington, D.C.: The Brookings Institution, 1964), p. 305.

[4]Council of Economic Advisers, *op. cit.,* p. 68.

the existence of the personal income taxes certainly became a greater obstacle to German growth with the passage of time.

The United States individual income tax, for a variety of reasons, does not seem to be such an obstacle to the growth of the economy as the British income taxes, although it has great importance as a source of revenue. As compared with the British, the American tax raises much more revenue from the lower and middle income classes and thus it ought to have less of an effect on personal savings and incentives. In 1963, the distribution of the revenues among the taxpayers was more even than that of any other country. Furthermore, the American nominal rates, when compared with those of the other countries, were comparatively low especially when the relative income method was used. It is apparent that the tax does not discriminate in favor of wages and salaries as the British tax does. Finally, the increase in the tax burden occurring between 1954 and 1963 was very small and was in part compensated by the decrease in the degree of erosion which occurred over the period. Thus, in conclusion, the United States tax cannot be assumed to have the same impact as the British and it should be considered relatively moderate, in spite of its substantial revenues.

In Italy and France the revenues from the personal income taxes were too small to play a significant role in the growth process of these economies. Furthermore, only a small part was collected from high income brackets or from incomes other than wages and salaries, so that the impact they may have had on personal savings or incentives must have been very marginal. In this connection it should be restated that the total tax burden of these two countries was very high, especially when it is related to per capita income; what was not collected from personal income taxes was collected from other taxes. These two countries as well as Japan may have been able to achieve higher growth rates at the cost of greater inequity.

Generally the European countries did not attempt to achieve a redistribution of income through progressive income taxation. Rather they had very extensive transfer payments programs which, together with high indirect taxes, can be considered as an alternative to progressive income taxation for redistribution. However, while progressive taxation has a tendency of transferring income from the higher to the lower income classes, the European method is more successful in transferring income from the middle to the lower income classes. This approach has some economic advantage since (a) the disincentive effects of the redistribution are much less significant; (b) much higher levels of personal savings become possible, and (c) the savings occur where they are more likely to be invested in more productive lines of activities rather than in residential construction. Against these economic advantages one must weigh the social costs connected with a system which is obviously inequitable.

BIBLIOGRAPHY

BOOKS

Barzini, Luigi. *The Italians.* New York: Bantam Books, Inc., 1965.

Beckerman, Wildred. *International Comparisons of Real Incomes.* Paris: O.E.C.D., 1966.

Bird, Richard, and Oldman, Oliver (eds.). *Readings on Taxation in Developing Countries.* Baltimore: The Johns Hopkins Press, 1964.

Clark, Colin. *Taxmanship.* London: Institute of Economic Affairs, 1964.

Cobb, Charles K., and Forte, Francesco. *Taxation in Italy.* "World Tax Series." Cambridge, Mass.: Harvard Law School, 1964.

Cosciani, Cesare. *Principii di Scienza delle Finanze.* Rome: Edizioni Ricerche, 1959.

Denison, Edward F. (assisted by Jean-Pierre Poullier). *Why Growth Rates Differ.* Washington, D.C.: The Brookings Institution, 1967.

Duberge, Jean. *The Social Psychology of Taxation in France Today.* Paris: 1961.

Duesenberry, James S. *Income, Saving and the Theory of Consumer Behavior.* Cambridge, Mass.: Harvard University Press, 1952.

Eckstein, Otto. *Public Finance.* Englewood Cliffs, N.J.: Prentice-Hall, Inc., 1964.

Einaudi, Luigi. *Saggi sul Risparmio e l'Imposta.* Torino: Giulio Einaudi Editore, 1958.

Friedman, Milton. *Theory of the Consumption Function.* Princeton: Princeton University Press, 1957.

Goode, Richard. *The Individual Income Tax.* Washington, D.C.: The Brookings Institution, 1964.

Grumpel, Henry J., and Boettcher, Carl. *Taxation in the Federal Republic of Germany.* "World Tax Series." Cambridge, Mass.: Harvard Law School, 1963.

Hayashi, Taizo. *Guide to Japanese Taxes.* Tokyo: Zaikei Shoho Sha, 1965.

Johansen, Leif. *Public Economics.* Amsterdam: North-Holland Publishing Company, 1965.

Johnston, J. *Econometric Methods.* New York: McGraw-Hill, 1963.

Kaldor, Nicholas. *An Expenditure Tax.* London: George Allen & Unwin Ltd, 1965.

Kindleberger, Charles P. *Europe's Postwar Growth: The Role of Labor Supply.* Cambridge, Mass.: Harvard University Press, 1967.

Kirschen, E., and others. *Economic Policy in Our Time.* 3 vols. Amsterdam: 1963 and 1964.

Lauré, Maurice. *Traité de Politique Fiscale.* Paris: P.U.F., 1957.

Lewis, Wilfred. *Federal Fiscal Policy in the Post-War Recessions.* Washington, D.C.: The Brookings Institution, 1962.

Maddison, Angus. *Economic Growth in the West.* New York: The Twentieth Century Fund, 1964.

Musgrave, Richard R. *The Theory of Public Finance.* New York: McGraw-Hill, 1959.

National Bureau of Economic Research and The Brookings Institution. *Foreign Tax Policies and Economic Growth.* New York: Columbia University Press, 1966.

———. *The Role of Direct and Indirect Taxes in the Federal Revenue System.* Princeton: Princeton University Press, 1964.

National Economic Development Council. *Conditions Favourable to Faster Growth.* London: 1963.

Norr, Martin, and Kerlan, Pierre. *Taxation in France.* "World Tax Series." Cambridge, Mass.: Harvard Law School, 1966.

Nortcliffe, E. B. *Common Market Fiscal Systems.* London: Sweet and Maxwell, 1960.

Ott, David J., and Ott, Attiat, F. *Federal Budget Policy.* Washington, D.C.: The Brookings Institution, 1964.

Pechman, Joseph A. *Federal Tax Policy,* Washington, D.C.: The Brookings Institution, 1966.

Pedone, Antonio. *Gettito Tributario e Congiuntura in Italia nel Periodo 1950-1962.* Rome: Istituto Nazionale per lo Studio della Congiuntura, 1965.

Plasschaert, Sylvain. *Taxable Capacity in Developing Countries.* Washington, D.C.: I.B.R.D. and I.D.A., Report No. Ec-103, 1962.

Répaci, Francesco A. *La Finanza Pubblica Italiana nel Secolo 1861-1960.* Bologna: Zanichelli Editore, 1962.

Rebout, L. *Systèmes Fiscaux et Marché Commun.* Paris: Ed. Sirey, 1961.

Reuss, Frederick, G. *Fiscal Policy for Growth without Inflation. The German Experience.* Baltimore: The Johns Hopkins Press, 1963.

Sarmet, Marcel. *L'Epargne dans le Marché Commun.* Paris: Editions Cujas, 1963.

Uematsu, Mario, and Coleman, Res. *Computation of Income in Japanese Income Taxation.* Cambridge, Mass.: Harvard Law School, 1963.

U.N.I.C.E. *Les Systèmes Fiscaux des Pays Membres de la Communauté Economique Européenne.* Brussels: 1960.

ARTICLES AND ESSAYS

Balassa, Bela. "The Purchasing-Power Parity Doctrine: A Reappraisal," *Journal of Political Economy,* December 1964.

Beard, T. R. "Progressive Income Taxation, Income Redistribution, and the Consumption Function," *National Tax Journal,* Vol. XIII, No. 2, June 1960.

Bird, Richard. "A Note on 'Tax Sacrifice' Comparisons," *National Tax Journal,* Vol. XVII, No. 3, September 1964.

Blackburn, John O. "Implicit Tax Rate Reductions with Growth, Progressive Taxes, Constant Progressivity, and a Fixed Public Share," *American Economic Review,* Vol. LVII, No. 1, March 1967.

Blancher, R. "Le Régime des Amortissements Fiscaux en France," *Revue de Science Financière,* No. 4, 1963.

Campet, Charles. "Les Systèmes Fiscaux des Pays de la Communauté Economique Européenne," *Revue de Science Financière,* No. 4, 1963.

Cohen, L. J. "An Empirical Measurement of the Built-in Flexibility of the Individual Income Tax," *American Economic Review,* May 1959.

_____."A More Recent Measurement of the Built-in Flexibility of the Individual Income Tax," *National Tax Journal,* June 1960.

Cosciani, Cesare. "Tax Reform in Italy: Hopes and Misgivings," *Banca Nazionale del Lavoro Quarterly Review,* September 1967.

Dosser, Douglas. "Tax Incidence and Growth," *Economic Journal,* Vol. LXXI, 1961.

_____."Incidence and Growth Further Considered," *Economic Journal,* Vol. LXXIII, 1963.

Duesenberry, James S., Eckstein, Otto, and Fromm, Gary. "A Simulation of the United States Economy in Recession," *Econometrica,* Vol. 28, October 1960.

Eckstein, Otto. "Indirect Versus Direct Taxes: Implications for Stability Investment," *Excise Tax Compendium,* Part I, Washington, D.C.: G.P.O., 1964.

Eckstein, Otto, assisted by Vito Tanzi. "Comparison of European and United States Tax Structures and Growth Implications," in N.B.E.R. and The Brookings Institution, *The Role of Direct and Indirect Taxes in the Federal Revenue System.* Princeton: Princeton University Press, 1964.

Flamant, M. "La Comparaison Internationale des Charges Fiscales et Parafiscales," *Revue de Science Financière,* No. 3, 1956.

Forte, Francesco. "Comment on Schedular and Global Income Taxes," in *Readings on Taxation in Developing Countries,* Richard Bird and Oliver Oldman (eds.). Baltimore: The Johns Hopkins Press, 1964.

Gantt, Andrew H. "Central Governments: Cash Deficits and Surpluses," *Review of Economics and Statistics,* February 1963.

Harberger, Arnold C. "Issues of Tax Reform for Latin America," in Organization of American States, *Fiscal Policy for Economic Growth in Latin America.* Baltimore: The Johns Hopkins Press, 1965.

Hicks, Ursula. "The Terminology of Tax Analysis," in *Readings in the Economics of Taxation,* Richard A. Musgrave and Carl S. Shoup (eds.). Homewood: R. D. Irwin, Inc., 1959.

_____."Direct Taxation and Economic Growth," *Oxford Economic Papers* (New Series), Vol. VIII, October 1956.

Houthakker, H. S. "An International Comparison of Personal Savings,"*International Statistical Bulletin* (Tokyo), May-June 1960.

International Bureau for Fiscal Documentation. "Taxation of Capital Gains Realized by Individuals in Europe," *European Taxation,* September 1965.

Kaldor, Nicholas. "Alternative Theories of Distribution," *Review of Economic Studies,* No. 62, 1955-56.

Kerlan, P. "Fiscalité et Marché Commun Européen," *Revue de Science Financière,* No. 1, 1959.

Knapp, John, and Lomax, Kenneth. "Britain's Growth Performance: The Enigma of the 1950's," *Lloyds Bank Review,* October 1964.

Kravis, Irving B., and Davenport, Michael W. S. "The Political Arithmetic of International Burden-Sharing," *The Journal of Political Economy,* Vol. LXXI, No. 4, August 1963.

Kullmer, Lore, "The Practical Significance of Tax Progressivity to the Value of the Yield Elasticity of a Tax," *Public Finance,* Vol. XX, Nos. 1-2, 1965.

_____."On the Yield Elasticity of a Progressive Income Tax in a Growing Economy," *Public Finance,* Vol. XX, Nos. 3-4, 1965.

"La Lira di Tutti." *Panorama,* November 1964.

Lansing, J. B., and Lydall, H. "An Anglo-American Comparison of Personal Saving," *Bulletin of the Oxford Institute of Statistics,* August 1960.

Laufenburger, V. H. "Problèmes fiscaux de l'épargne individuelle de l'autofinancement, de l'amortissement," *Revue de Science Financière,* April-June 1965.

Lauré, Maurice. "Impôts et Productivité," *Productivité Française,* No. 17, May 1953.

_____. "Influence de la Fiscalité sur la Formation de l'Epargne," *Revue de Science Financière,* April-June 1954.

La Volpe, G. "La Previdenza Sociale nella Formazione del Reddito Nazionale: Evoluzione Recente e Prospettive in Italia (1956-1970)," *Giornale degli Economisti,* November-December 1963.

Mishan, E. J., and Dicks-Mireaux, L. A. "Progressive Taxation in an Inflationary Economy," *American Economic Review,* September 1958.

Musgrave, R. A., and Miller, M. H. "Built-in Flexibility," *American Economic Review,* Vol. 38, No. 1, March 1948.

_____. "Effects of Tax Policy on Private Capital Formation," in *Fiscal and Debt Management Policies,* Research Studies for the Commission on Money and Credit. Englewood Cliffs, N.J.: Prentice Hall, 1963.

Needleman, L. "The Burden of Taxation: An International Comparison," *National Institute Economic Review,* No. 14, March 1961.

Parent, J. "Impôt Pregressif, Matière Fiscale et Croissance Economique," *Revue de Science Financière*, No. 3, 1956.

Peacock, Alan T. "Built-in Flexibility and Economic Growth," in *Stabile Preise in Wachsender Wirtschaft*, Bombach Gottfried, (ed.). Tubingen: J. C. B. Mohr, 1960.

Pearse, P. H. "Automatic Stabilization and the British Taxes on Income," *Review of Economic Studies*, February 1962.

Pechman, J. A. "Erosion of the Individual Income Tax," *National Tax Journal*, Vol. 10, No. 1, March 1957.

____. "Yield of the Individual Income Tax during a Recession," in *Policies to Combat Depressions*. Princeton: Princeton University Press, 1956.

Pottier, P. "Fiscalité et Croissance dans le IVe Plan," *Revue de Science Financière*, No. 2, 1964.

Prest, A. R. "The Sensitivity of the Yield of Personal Income Tax in the United Kingdom," *The Economic Journal*, September 1962.

Reid, G. L. "Social Security in Britain and the Six," *The Banker*, June 1963.

Rey, Mario. "Estimating Tax Evasions: The Example of the Italian General Sales Tax," *Public Finance*, Vol. XX, Nos. 3-4, 1965.

Sarcinelli, Mario. "The Overall Direct Tax Rate on Earned Incomes in Italy," *Banca Nazionale del Lavoro Quarterly Review*, September 1967.

Shoup, Carl S. "Comparative Approaches to Tax Policy within the Major Countries," National Tax Association, *Proceedings*, 1965.

Solomon, Robert. "The Full Employment Budget Surplus as an Analytical Concept" (paper presented at Annual Meeting of American Statistical Association), Minneapolis, September 8, 1962.

Tanzi, Vito. "Comparing International Tax Burdens: A Suggested Method," *Journal of Political Economy*, October 1968.

Tanzi, Vito. "A Proposal for a Dynamically Self-Adjusting Individual Income Tax," *Public Finance*, Vol. 4, 1966.

Tanzi, Vito. "La Struttura del Sistema Fiscale Italiano: Un Confronto Internazionale," *Rivista Internazionale di Scienze Economiche e Commerciali*, Anno XIII, No. 6, 1966.

Weckstein, Richard S. "Fiscal Reform and Economic Growth," *National Tax Journal*, December 1964.

REPORTS

France

Bulletin de Documentation Pratique des Impôts Directs et des Droits d'Enregistrement. Paris: Editions Francis Lefèbvre, 32e année, No. 5, May 1966.

France, Direction Générale des Impôts. "Comparaison entre les Charges Fiscales Françaises et Américaines." Paris: no date.

France. Institut National de le Statistique et des Etudes Economiques. *Tableaux de L'Economie Française*. Paris: 1966.

France. Ministère de l'Economie et des Finances. *Statistiques et Etudes Financières.* Paris: Imprimerie Nationale, monthly.
_____. *Statistiques et Etudes Financières,* Supplément. Paris: Imprimerie Nationale, monthly.
_____. *Renseignements Statistiques Relatifs aux Impôts Directs.* Paris: Imprimerie National, 76e année Exercice 1965.

Germany

Germany. Deutsche Bundesbank. *Monthly Report.* Frankfurt.
Germany. Federal Office of Statistics. *Statistical Yearbook, 1966.* West Baden, 1966.

Italy

Associazione fra le Società Italiane per Azioni. *Le Finanze Publiche dei sei Paesi della C.E.E. nel 1957.* Rome: 1958.
Cosciani, Cesare. *Stato dei Lavori della Commissione per lo Studio della Riforma Tributaria.* Milan: Giuffré, 1964.
Gazzetta Ufficiale della Republica Italiana. Rome: Libreria dello Stato.
Italy. Istituto Centrale di Statistica. *Annuario Statistico Italiano.* Rome: Istituto Poligrafico dello Stato.
Italy. Ministero delle Finanze. *Annuario Statistico Finanziario,* Vol. 5. Rome: Istituto Poligrafico dello Stato, 1964.
_____. *L'Attività Tributaria dal 1954 al 1964,* Vols. I and II. Rome: Istituto Poligrafico dello Stato, 1964.
_____. *L'Attività Tributaria nel 1965.* Rome: Istituto Poligrafico dello Stato, 1966.
Supplemento al Bollettino Ufficiale delle Imposte Dirette. Rome: Istituto Poligrafico dello Stato.
Unione Italiana Camere Commercio Industria Agricoltura. *Compendio Economico Italiano.* Rome: Giuffré, 1963.

Japan

Japan. Economic Planning Agency. *Japanese Economic Statistics.* Tokyo: monthly.
Japan. Ministry of Finance. Budget Bureau. *The Budget in Brief.* Tokyo: 1964.
Japan. Ministry of Finance. Tax Bureau. *Major Statistics of Taxation in Japan* (available only in Japanese). Tokyo: 1965.
An Outline of Japanese Taxes. Tokyo: annual.
Japan. Ministry of Foreign Affairs. *Statistical Survey of Economy of Japan.* Tokyo: annual.
Japan. Prime Minister's Office. Bureau of Statistics. *Survey of Trends in Saving for 1960 and 1961.* Tokyo.

United Kingdom

Great Britain. Board of Inland Revenue. *Report of the Commissioners of Her Majesty's Inland Revenue.* London: H.M.S.O., annual.
Great Britain. British Information Services. *The British System of Taxation.* London, 1965.
Great Britain. Central Statistical Office. *New Contributions to Economic Statistics,* Studies in Official Statistics, No. 10. London: H.M.S.O., 1964.
____. *National Income and Expenditure.* London: H.M.S.O., 1966.
____. *Economic Trends,* annual.
Great Britain. *Report of the Committee on Turnover Taxation.* London: H.M.S.O., 1964.

United States

U.S. Advisory Commission on Intergovernmental Relations. *Measures of State and Local Fiscal Capacity and Tax Effort.*
U.S. Committee on Ways and Means. *Excise Tax Compendium,* Part I and II. Washington, D.C.: G.P.O., 1964.
U.S. Congress. Joint Economic Committee. *The Federal Tax System: Facts and Problems, 1964.* Washington, D.C.: G.P.O., 1964.
____. Economic Policies and Practices, Paper No. 3. *A Description and Analysis of Certain European Capital Markets.* Washington, D.C.: G.P.O., 1964.
U.S. Council of Economic Advisers. *Economic Report of the President.* Annual. Washington, D.C.,: G.P.O.
U.S. Department of Commerce. *Statistical Abstract of the United States.* Washington, D.C.,: G.P.O., 1966.
U.S. Internal Revenue Service. *Statistics of Income.* Washington, D.C., G.P.O., 1966.

Others

Communauté Economique Européenne. *Rapport du Comité Fiscal et Financier (Neumark Report).* Brussels: 1962.
European Economic Community. *General Statistical Bulletin.* Brussels: monthly.
Gilbert, Milton, and associates. *Comparative National Products and Price Levels.* O.E.E.C.: 1958.
Gilbert, Milton, and Kravis, Irving B. *An International Comparison of National Products and the Purchasing Power of Currencies.* O.E.E.C.: 1964.
International Bureau of Fiscal Documentation. *European Taxation.* Holland: bimonthly.
O.E.C.D. *National Accounts Statistics, 1954-1964.* Paris: March 1966.

INDEX

British surtax: background, 19; rates, 20; reforms, 20; revenues, 70-71

Burdens, income tax: absolute income method, 24-25; alternative measures, 45-49; erosion, 86-87, 87t; per capita income, 22-24; relative income method, 31-34

Business income, treatment of: France, 56, 57t, 58t, 59; Germany, 62; Italy, 65-66; Japan, 72-73, 73t; U.K., 69-70, 70t

Capital gains tax: France, 7, 10; Germany, 12; Italy, 15; Japan, 16; U.K., 20

Complementary tax: French, 10; Italian, 15

Cyclical behavior of tax: France, 90-91; Germany, 93-95; Italy, 96-98; Japan, 101-3; U.K., 104-5; U.S., 105

Deductions and exemptions: France, 8-9; Germany, 11-12, 92t; Italy, 15; Japan, 16, 100t; U.K., 18-19

Denison, Edward F., 123

Distribution of income: See Income distribution

Dosser, 90

Economic growth: American taxes, 105-9; British taxes, 103-5; French taxes, 89-91; German taxes, 91-95; Italian taxes, 95-98; Japanese taxes, 98-103; tax systems, 1-3, 123-26

Effective tax rates: 76t; France, 56-60, 60t; Germany, 61-62, 61t, 62t; Italy, 66-69, 67t, 69t; Japan, 71-74, 72t, 73t; U.K., 70-71, 71t

Einkommensteuer, 11, 40

Elasticity and flexibility: American taxes, 106-9; British taxes, 103-5, 104t; French taxes, 89-90, 90t; German taxes, 93, 93t, 95t; Italian taxes, 95-96, 96t; Japanese taxes, 98-103, 103t

Erosion, tax: compared, 78t, 80t; defined, 77; France, 56, 57t, 80-81, 85; Germany, 62, 81, 84; Italy, 65-66, 79, 81, 85-86; Japan, 72-74, 81, 84-85; specific incomes, 80-81; tax burdens, 86-87; trends, 84-86, 85t; U.S., 78, 81

Evasion: general, 54, 81-84; Germanic countries, 83; Italy, 66-69; Latin countries, 83

Families, treatment of: compared, 26t; France, 9; Germany, 11-12; Italy, 15; Japan, 16; U.K., 19; U.S., 26t

Flexibility: See Elasticity and flexibility

Goode, Richard, 7, 107, 116

Growth: See Economic growth

Häuser, Karl, 114

Houthakker, H. S., 120

I.G.E. (Italian General Sales Tax), 5; Evasion, 83

Imposta Complementare, 15, 40, 69, 85-86

Income brackets, 38-44

Income distribution: functional, 51t; individual, 51t

Italian general sales tax: See I.G.E.

Italian schedular taxes, 14-15, 64-69

Kaldor, Nicholas, 112

Komiya, Ryutaro, 115

135

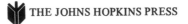 THE JOHNS HOPKINS PRESS

Designed by Arlene J. Sheer

Composed in Press Roman text and display by Jones Composition Company, Inc.

Printed on 60-lb. Perkins and Squier R by Universal Lithographers, Inc.

Bound in Columbia Riverside Linen by L.H. Jenkins Co., Inc.